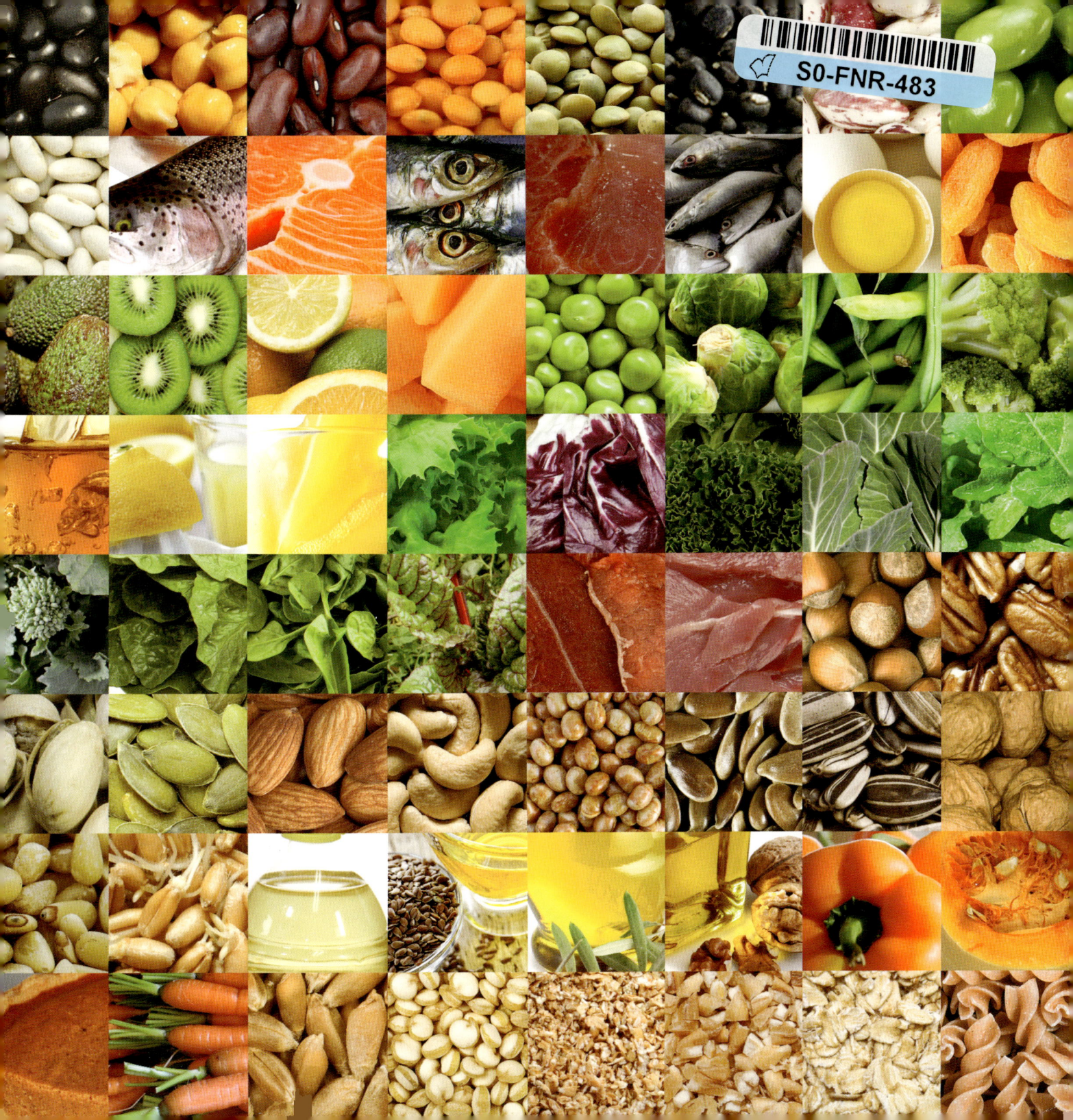

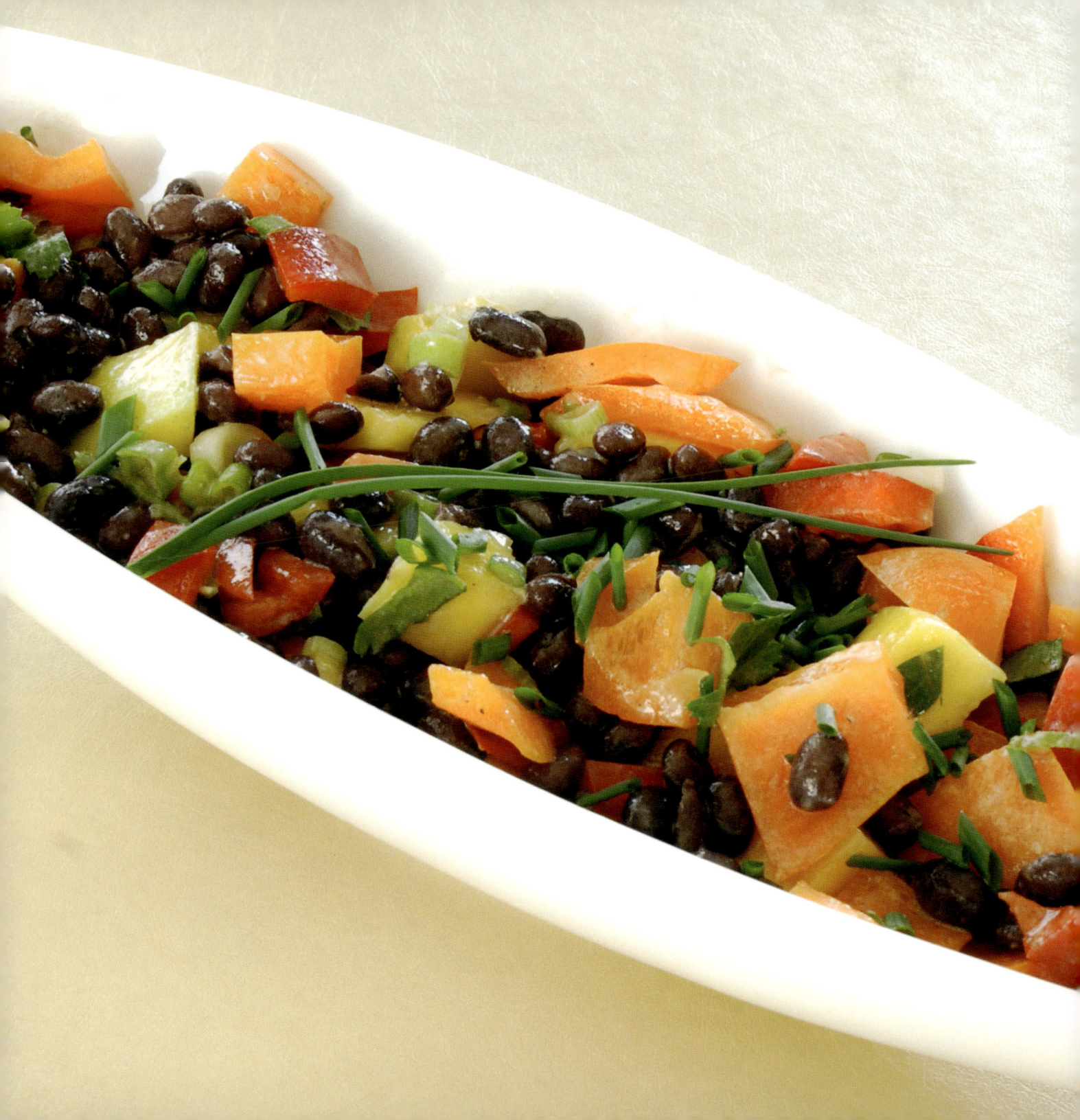

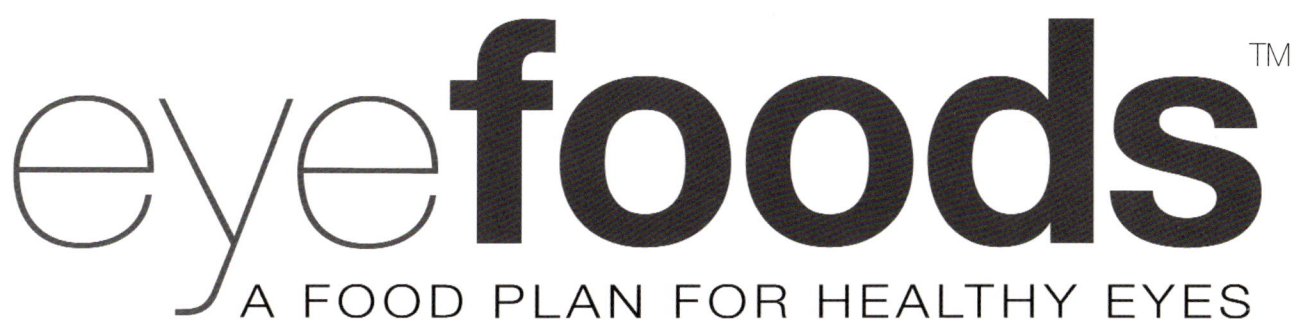

eyefoods™
A FOOD PLAN FOR HEALTHY EYES

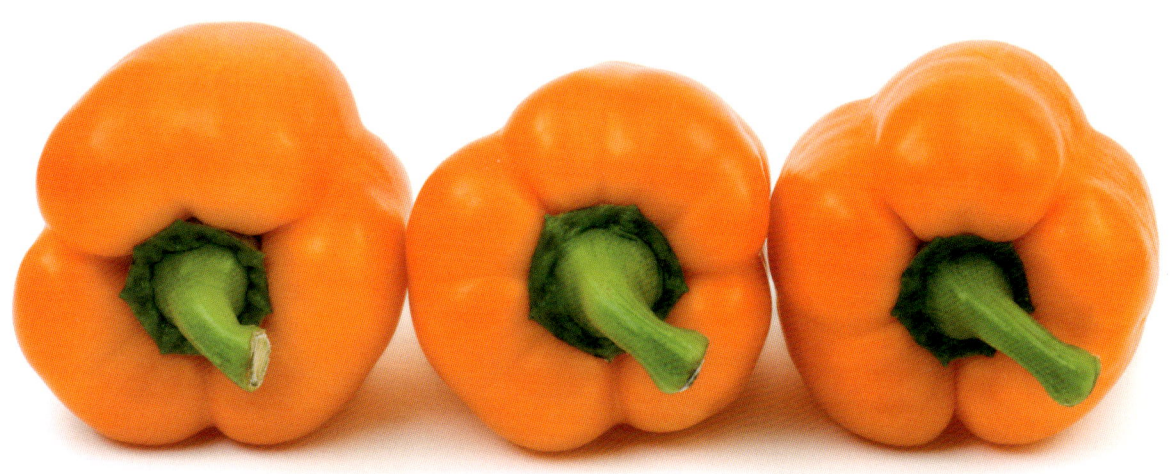

DR. LAURIE CAPOGNA, OD & DR. BARBARA PELLETIER, OD
www.eyefoods.com

LB Media Concepts Inc.

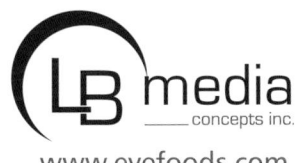

www.eyefoods.com

Developed by: LB Media Concepts
Editorial: Erin Knight
Design: Rose Gowsell-Pattison, Plan B Graphic Design
Consultant: Elizabeth Shaver Heeney MEd, MSc, RD

Photographs: Laurie Capogna: p. 30; Robert Nowell: backcover, p. 5, p. 6; Barbara Pelletier: p. 2, p.8, p.12, p. 14 (top), p. 28, p. 47, p. 55, p. 63, p. 68, p. 70, p. 73, p. 82, p. 83, p. 88, p. 98, p. 118, p. 130, p. 137 (middle left, middle right), p. 141; Shutterstock: 54613: p. 59; Africa Studio: p. 117; Andrjuss: p. 93; Robert Anthony: p. 102; Barri: p. 74; Don Bendickson: p. 60; BestImagesEver.com: p. 123; Bork: p. 44; Bruce Amos: p. 19; Barbro Bergfeldt: p. 106; Ilker Canikligil: p. 110; Anna Chelnokova: p. 64; Chiyacat: p. 18, p. 104; Sharon Day: p. 81, p. 91, p. 98, p. 107, p. 111 (bottom); George Dolgikh: p. 113; Olesya Dorozhenko: p. 89; Igor Dutina: p. 27, p. 52, p. 58, p. 90; Elena Elisseeva: p. 41, p. 107 (top); Brooke Fuller: p. 100; Gelpi: p. 24; Givaga: p. 32; Gordan Gledec: p. 103; Jiri Hera: p. 21, p. 75; Patrick Hermans: p. 69 (bottom); Margrit Hirsch: p. 54; Ivanova Inga: p. 49 (bottom); Levent Konuk: p. 39; Yuriy Kulyk: p. 115; Karin Hildebrand Lau: p. 76; Olga Lyubkina: p. 92; Matin: p. 127, p. 129, pp. 131-133, p. 138, p. 140; Monkey Business Images: p. 84; Naluwan: p. 112; Nayashkova Olga: p. 94; Noma: p. 79; Nordling: p. 97 (top); Patty Orly: p. 111 (right); Tatiana Popova: Cover, p. 3; Alexander Raths: p. 35; David Reilly: p. 25, p. 48 (top); Josh Resnick: p. 85; Rodho: p. 86; Elena Schweitzer: p. 53; Sobur: p. 77; David P. Smith: p. 91; Stargazer: p. 96; Tanatat: p. 95; Tatniz: p. 120; Tish1: p. 50; VLDR: p. 61; Valentyn Volkov: p. 109; Denis Vrublevski: p. 121; Ivonne Wierink: p. 70; Wiktory: p. 78; Wutthichai: p. 56; Lisa F. Young: p. 51; Tania Zbrodko: p. 36; Dusan Zidar: p. 108

Library and Archives Canada Cataloging in Publication

Capogna, Laurie
    Eyefoods: a food plan for healthy eyes / Laurie Capogna, Barbara Pelletier.

Includes bibliographical references and index.
ISBN 978-0-9868079-0-9

    1. Eye--Diseases--Diet therapy.
2. Eye--Diseases--Prevention. I. Pelletier, Barbara
II. Title.

RE991.C36 2011   617.7'0654   C2011-900232-9

Copyright © 2011 LB MEDIA CONCEPTS. All rights reserved. No part of this publication may be reproduced, stored in a retrieval system or be transmitted in any form or by any means, electronic, mechanical, photocopying, recording, or otherwise, without the prior written permission of LB Media Concepts.

This book has been written for informational purposes only. The contents are based upon the research and observations of the authors, and every effort has been made to ensure the accuracy of the contents as of the date published. Readers are of course encouraged to confirm the information contained herein with other sources. Readers should also consult with their own professional health care provider with respect to any specific recommendations, as the information contained in this book is not intended to replace client specific medical advice. The authors and the publisher expressly disclaim responsibility for any adverse effects arising from the use of application of the information contained in this book.

Printed and bound in Canada

About the authors

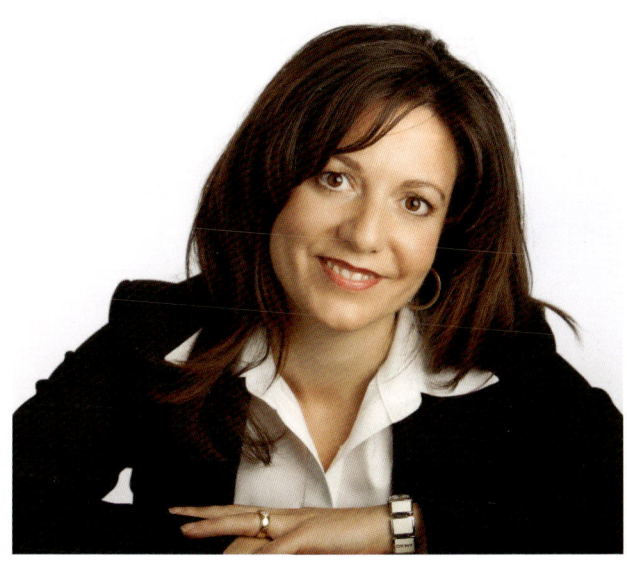

Dr. Laurie Capogna
Optometrist

Dr. Laurie Capogna graduated from the University of Waterloo in Ontario, Canada with her Doctor of Optometry degree in 1998. She has been practicing optometry since 1998, with an interest in ocular health and refractive surgery. Dr. Capogna is an active partner in Peninsula Eye Associates, where she provides full-spectrum optometric care in a surgical eye care center.

In 2009, Dr. Capogna started a Low Vision Clinic where she helps patients with eye disease and vision loss to achieve their daily goals. Dr. Capogna practices comprehensive optometry where she focuses on all three aspects of eye care, including prevention, treatment and rehabilitation.

In addition to practicing at Peninsula Eye Associates, Dr. Capogna was a founding optometrist of *Lasik Provision*, where she provides pre- and post-operative care to refractive surgery patients. She is a member of the College of Optometrists of Ontario, the Ontario Association of Optometrists, the Canadian Association of Optometrists, and the Ocular Nutrition Society.

During her optometric career, Dr. Capogna has had a keen interest in the relationship between nutrition and the prevention of eye disease, and has treated thousands of patients. Her quest to help these patients prevent the progression of eye disease and maintain eye health led her to research the area of nutrition and eye health. It is through her daily interactions with patients that she saw the need for a way to educate people regarding the benefits of good nutrition and vision.

In her free time, Dr. Capogna enjoys cooking and entertaining for friends and family. Her parents immigrated to Canada from Italy in the 1950s, and she was raised on a fruit and greenhouse farm in southwestern Ontario. Her Italian heritage and experience with growing fruits and vegetables has nurtured her interest in nutrition and cooking. She strives to use local ingredients in her meals and loves to incorporate cooking techniques from her Italian heritage.

Dr. Capogna has worked with her partner and friend, Dr. Barbara Pelletier, for over ten years in Niagara Falls, Ontario. They have always shared a common interest in nutrition and cooking. Through their many conversations regarding patient care and the prevention of eye disease, the topics of nutrition and eye health were always a common theme. These conversations were the genesis of *Eyefoods™: A Food Plan for Healthy Eyes*.

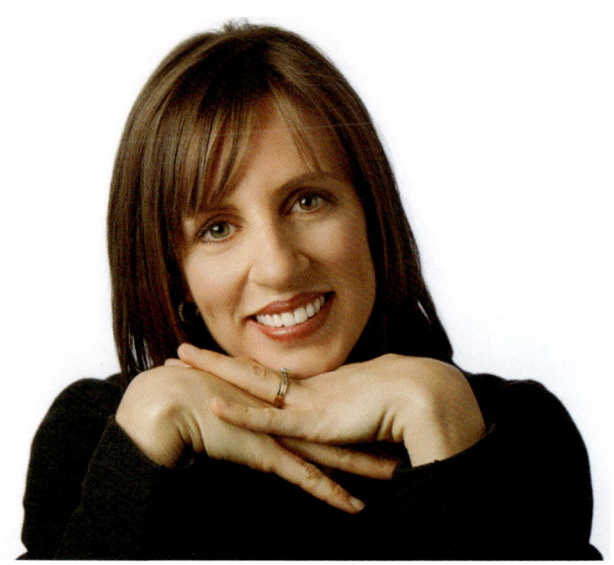

Dr. Barbara Pelletier
Optometrist

Dr. Barbara Pelletier was born in Jonquière, Québec. She graduated and received her Doctor of Optometry degree from the Université de Montréal in 1998. After practicing in the Ottawa, Ontario area, she moved to the Niagara Peninsula. Dr. Pelletier is an active partner at Iris Optometrists in Welland, Ontario with her husband, Dr. Christian Nanini, where she practices comprehensive optometry. She also has extensive experience in laser refractive surgery management, providing patients with pre- and post-operative care as part of Dr. Andrew Taylor's team since 2000. She is a member of the College of Optometrists of Ontario, the Ontario Association of Optometrists, l'Association des optométristes du Québec, the Canadian Association of Optometrists, and the Ocular Nutrition Society.

She has been interested in nutrition for many years now and loves learning new recipes to include healthy foods for her family's diet. Since a lot of her patients have eye diseases and inquire about what to eat to maintain healthier eyes, she had a dream of finding a way to raise awareness about how to get all the necessary nutrients through fresh ingredients.

She has been practicing photography since her teenage years and has done some of the photos you will see in this book. She also has a passion for playing the flute and for fitness. She practices yoga regularly and enjoys hiking, biking, and tennis playing.

Elizabeth Shaver Heeney MEd, MSc, RD

Elizabeth Shaver Heeney MEd, MSc, RD worked as a consultant for *Eyefoods™: A Food Plan for Healthy Eyes.* She is a graduate of the University of Western Ontario and the University of Guelph. She is a registered dietitian with over 20 years of experience in public health nutrition. In addition, she is a teacher, consultant, researcher, and author. She is a member of the College of Dietitians of Ontario, Dietitians of Canada, and the Ontario Society of Nutrition Professionals in Public Health.

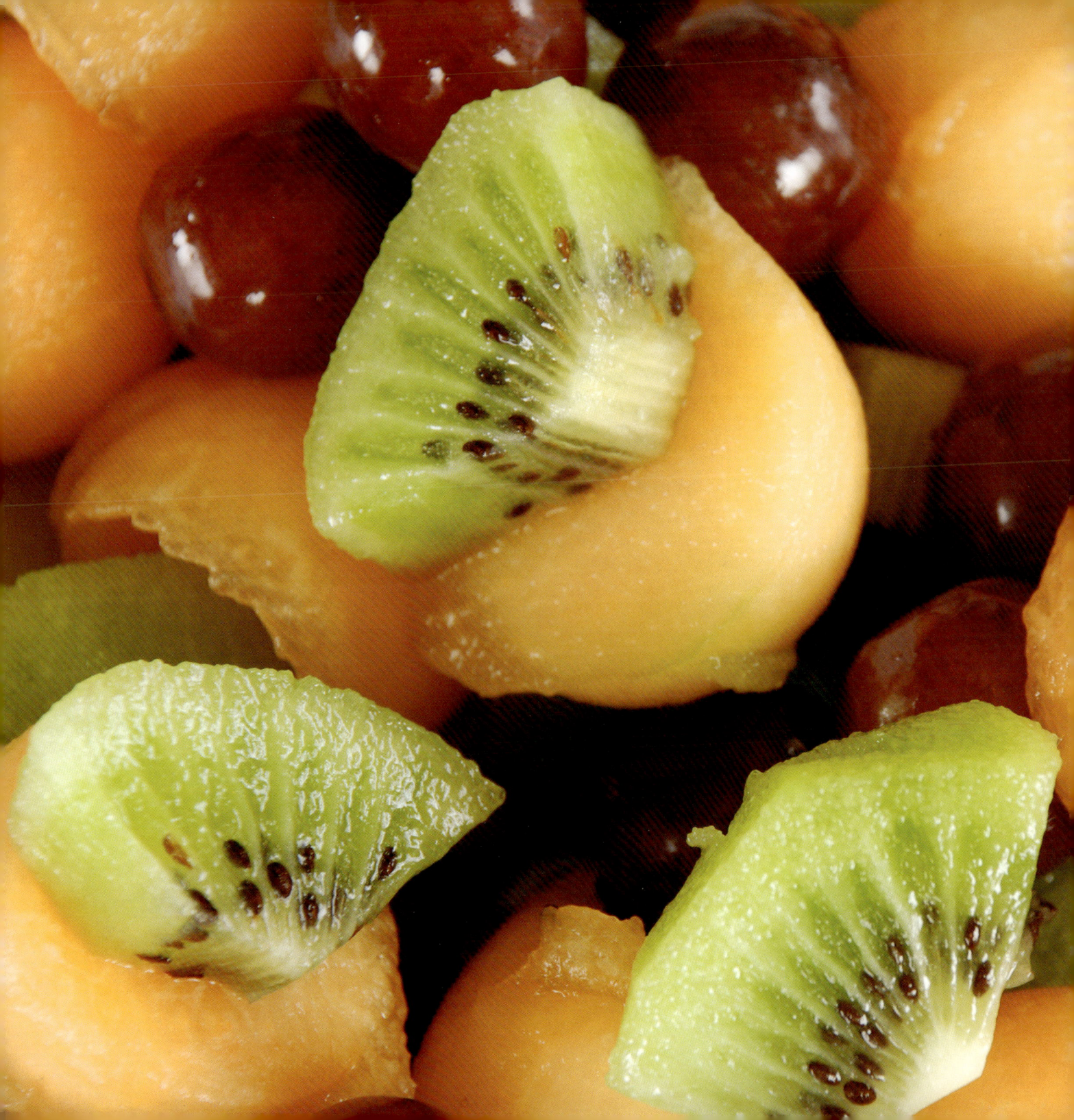

This book is dedicated to our patients.

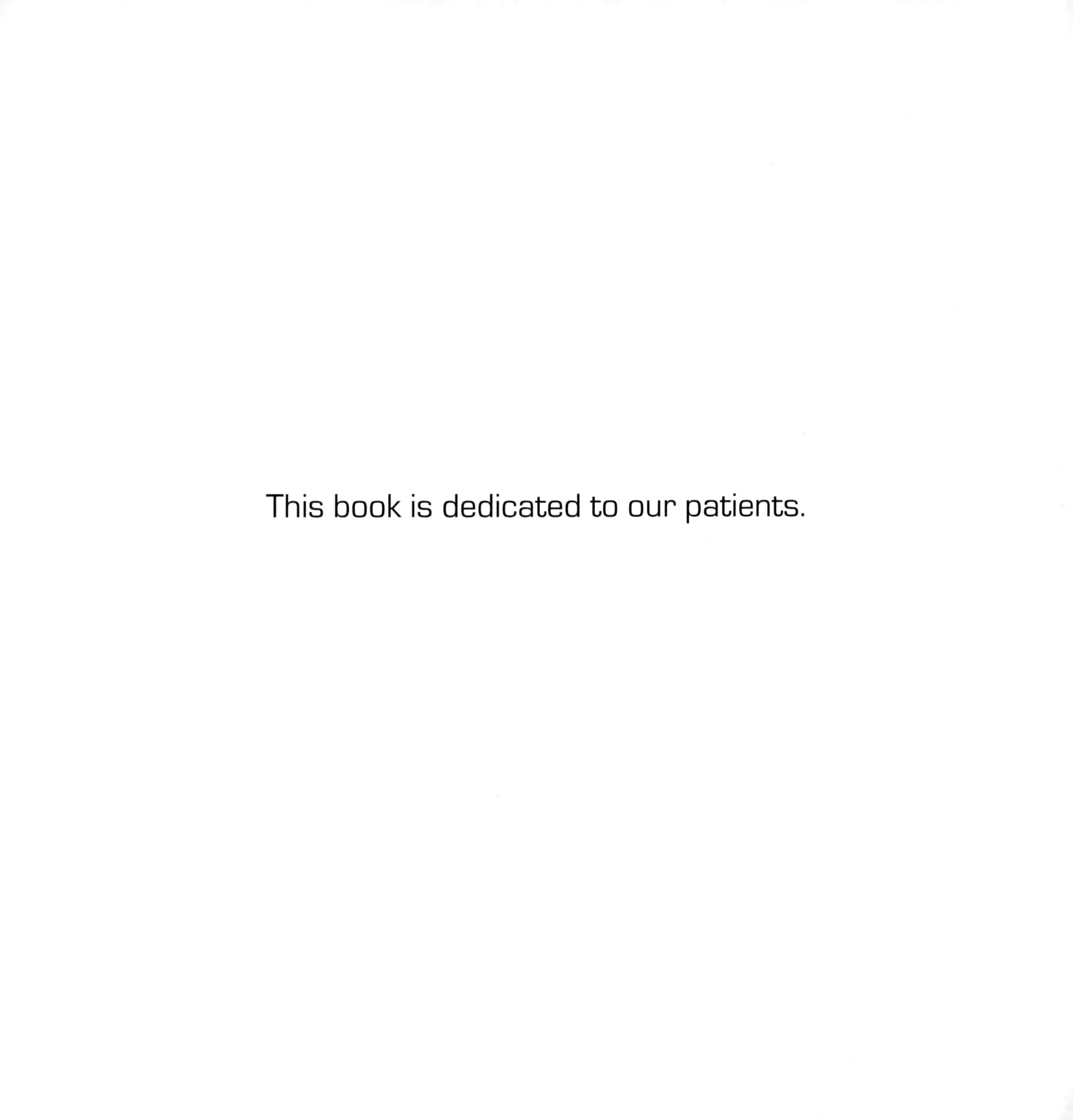

Table of Contents

Forewords 14
Introduction 19

Part One: The Basics

Chapter One: Eye Health and Disease 25
    Age-Related Macular Degeneration
    Cataracts
    Dry Eye Syndrome
    Eyelid Disorders

Chapter Two: Eye Nutrients 49
    Antioxidants
    Lutein and Zeaxanthin
    Vitamin C
    Omega-3 Fatty Acids
    Vitamin E
    Zinc
    Beta-Carotene
    Vitamin D
    Fiber
    Glycemic Index and Glycemic Load

Part Two: The Details

Chapter Three: Eyefoods 69
    Leafy Green Vegetables
    Cold Water Fish
    Orange Vegetables
    Orange Peppers
    Green Vegetables

Eggs
　　　Fruit and Juice
　　　Lean Protein
　　　Nuts and Seeds
　　　Whole Grains
　　　Beans and Lentils
　　　Flax Seed
　　　Oil

Chapter Four: Lifestyle and General Health 113
　　　UV Exposure
　　　Smoking
　　　Body Mass Index and Waist Circumference
　　　Physical Activity
　　　Age-Related Macular Degeneration and Cardiovascular Disease

Part Three: The Plan

Chapter Five: The Eyefoods Plan 127
　　　Weekly Targets
　　　Serving Sizes
　　　The Eyefoods Nutrition Plan
　　　Track It
　　　The Eyefoods Lifestyle Plan

Eyefood for Thought................ 138
Acknowledgements 140
Glossary 142
Notes 152
References 158
Index 167

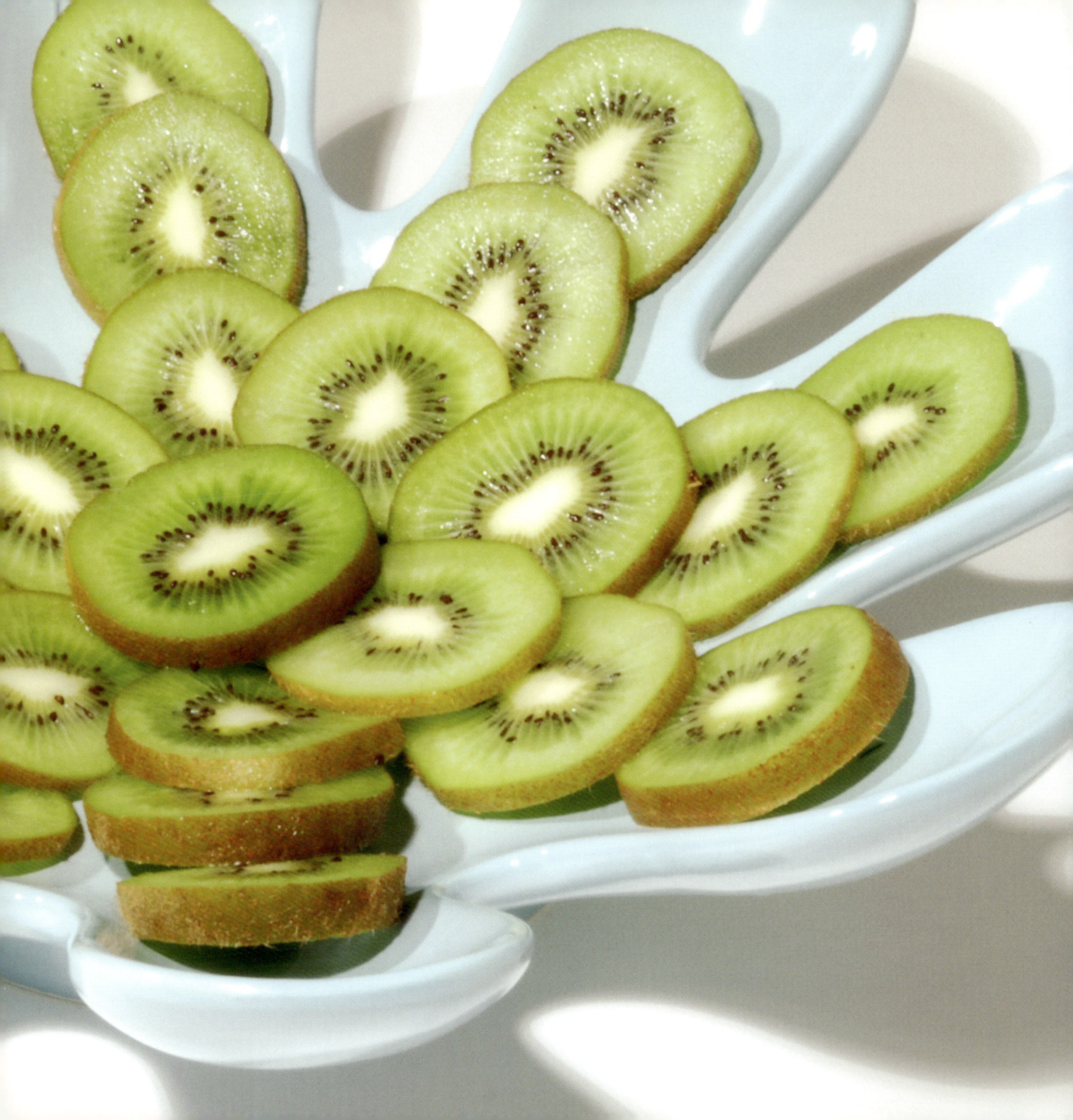

As eye doctors, we have seen the effects that eye disease can have on our patients' lives. Many people don't realize that the choices they make can help to preserve their vision. Our mission is to empower our patients and the public with the knowledge they need to prevent eye disease and vision loss.

Forewords

Our vision is our most precious gift. It is the one sense people are most eager to preserve their entire life. Everyday, as optometrists, we educate our patients about this. Prescribing the correct lifestyle habits is as essential as prescribing the best products and professional services. Current science proves everyday the close link between vision and diet. As passionate optometrists, Dr. Capogna and Dr. Pelletier are committed to popularize the scientific information and educate us through our diets. The joy of eating and science together in the same book. Let this book be your guide as it will help you experience better vision.

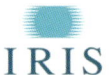
**Dr. Francis Jean, OD, President
IRIS, The Visual Group**

This is an important and timely book. As a population, the human race is currently under the greatest environment assault in recorded time; both from toxins that we are exposed to on a daily basis and from the fundamental changes to our daily nutritional intake from our food supply. In 2001, the Age-Related Eye Disease Study sponsored by the National Eye Institute, confirmed what we as clinicians have intuitively known by confirming the important role of nutrition in maintaining eyesight and reducing the risk of developing advanced age-related macular degeneration. Since the time of this clinical trial, there has been an explosion of study and interest into the components of nutrition and lifestyle that maintain healthy ocular function. This book builds on these bodies of work.

I have had the pleasure of knowing and working professionally with Drs. Laurie Capogna and Barbara Pelletier for over ten years. In my 15 year career as an anterior segment and refractive ophthalmic surgeon, I have worked closely with numerous medical professionals and these two doctors stand out for their clinical inquisitiveness, their thoroughness, and their caring attention to the well being of their patients. These attributes are well reflected in their crafting of this book. Throughout our collective careers, our understanding of the multitude of benefits from informed nutritional and lifestyle choices have been borne out.

I am fortunate and honored to introduce their first book, which recognizes their leading role in the fields of nutrition and lifestyle as they apply to ocular disease. It is concisely written and beautifully photographed. The contents are easily translated into daily lifestyle choices. For patients and clinicians alike, this book will serve as an excellent reference source for these important topics. This is the first work from two authors whose voices I am sure we will continue to hear from again.

Andrew W. Taylor, MD, FRCS(C), Dip. ABO.

Forewords

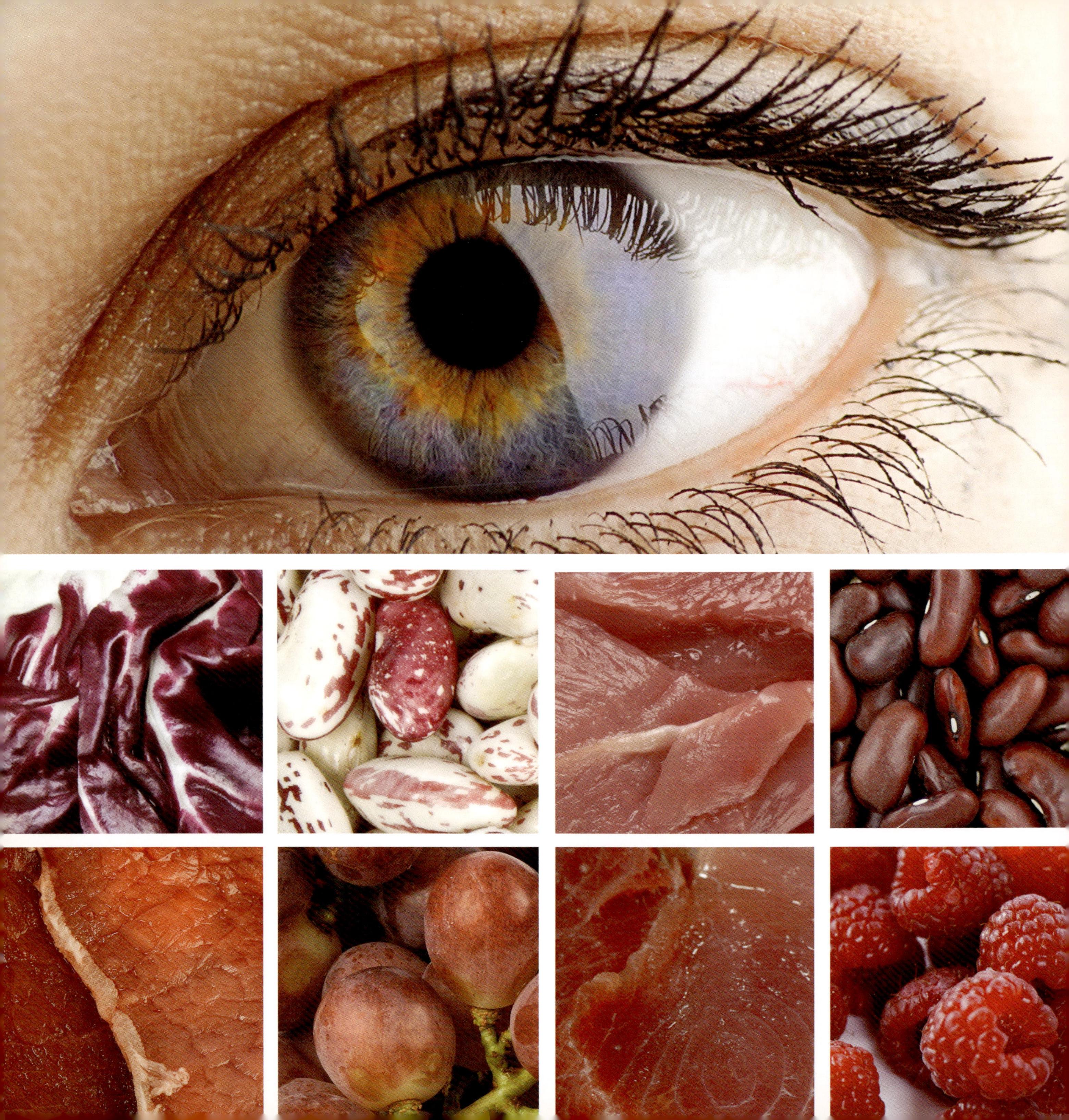

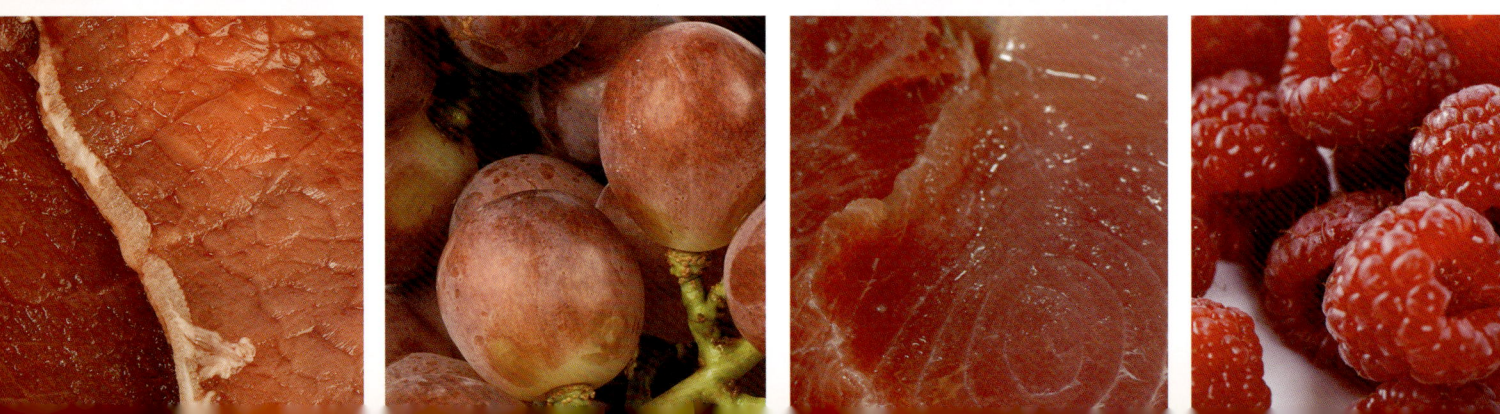

Introduction

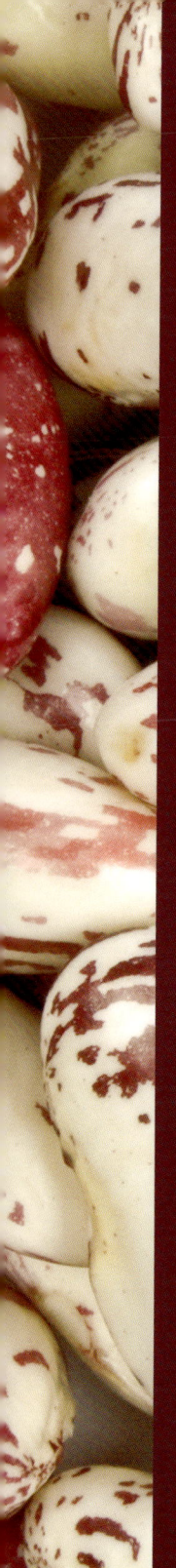

This book is for everyone who wants to learn more about eye health and the prevention of eye disease. We have taken the experience we have gained in our combined 25 years of practice, integrated it with the most up-to-date scientific research, and created *Eyefoods: A Food Plan for Healthy Eyes.*

Keep this book handy, and browse through it frequently. You will learn something new each time you pick it up.

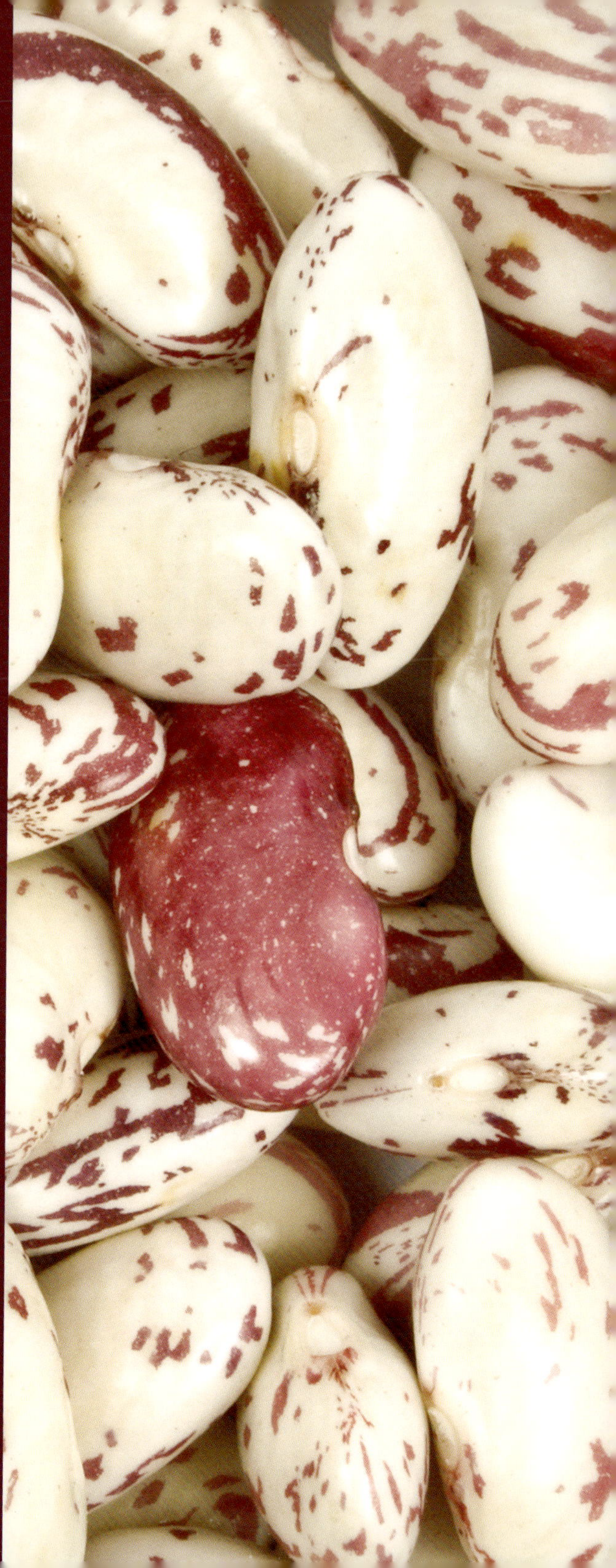

Introduction

Our environment, our habits, and especially the foods that we eat have significant impacts on every aspect of our health. Though it can be easy to take good vision for granted, following a diet designed with eye health in mind is the best way to prevent eye disease and possible vision loss.

As optometrists, we became particularly excited about the power of certain foods to prevent eye disease. We began incorporating foods that have powerful healing or disease-preventing properties, known as *nutraceuticals*, into our families' diets. Still, we wanted to develop a tool to encourage our patients and the public to discover nutraceuticals for themselves. Developed over months of research, this book is that tool. It is a plan for preventing eye disease and maintaining eye health through the power of food.

With *Eyefoods: A Food Plan for Healthy Eyes*, we strive to increase public awareness by sharing scientifically proven information.

Everyone will benefit from adding eyefoods to their diet. Whether you have an existing eye condition or are trying to maintain healthy eyes, the recommendations made in this book will help you preserve your vision.

The basic principle behind eyefoods is that these foods are full of the nutrients essential to eye health. These are eye nutrients. After careful review of scientific studies, we have determined the most important nutrients for the prevention of eye disease and the promotion of eye health. Each of these nutrients helps decrease the risk of eye disease, either on its own or in conjunction with other nutrients. In addition to promoting eyefoods, we focus on other important lifestyle factors such as non-smoking, exercise, and UV protection. This book is organized to provide you with the necessary knowledge for making the food and lifestyle choices that will preserve your eye health.

The Basics: Chapter 1, "Eye Health and Disease," and Chapter 2, "Eye Nutrients," discuss basic principles and explain the relationship between eye disease and good nutrition. Chapter 1 and Chapter 2 make up the foundation of the eyefoods plan.

The Details: Chapter 3, "Eyefoods," and Chapter 4, "Lifestyle and General Health," provide you with details regarding the food and lifestyle choices that will directly improve your eye health.

The Plan: Chapter 5, "The Eyefoods Plan" outlines an easy-to-follow method of integrating eyefoods and the eyefoods lifestyle recommendations into your life.

Frequently Asked Questions:

Doctor, what can I do to help my vision?
We hear this question on a regular basis in our offices. We tell our patients that eating nutrient-dense foods and following an eye-friendly lifestyle will provide them with the building blocks for good vision.

Are nutrients and eye disease related?
Through careful review of scientific studies, we have discovered that certain food nutrients play an important role in preventing many common eye diseases and vision problems. We have established weekly targets for foods dense in eye nutrients, which we have labeled *eyefoods*.

Which nutrients promote eye health?
Of all the nutrients necessary for eye

health, lutein and zeaxanthin, which are carotenoids, are the most important. Omega-3 fatty acids are also highly important. Cold-water fish such as sardines and salmon, as well as flax seeds, contain various types of omega-3 fatty acids. Antioxidants such as vitamin C, vitamin E, and beta-carotene also help maintain eye health. Many fruits and vegetables are high in lutein and zeaxanthin and antioxidants.

Which foods should I eat?
Certain fruits and vegetables, whole grains, and fish are best. Scientific studies have shown that the nutrients found in these foods can help prevent or slow the progression of eye diseases such as age-related macular degeneration, cataracts and dry eye syndrome.[1]

How can I add these foods to my diet?
If you follow the eyefoods plan outlined in this book, you will be consuming the appropriate foods to help preserve your eye health.

Do eyefoods have other health benefits?
Studies show that these foods also help to prevent certain cancers and heart disease. Adding eyefoods to your diet will protect your vision and improve your overall health and well-being.[2]

Who will benefit from eating eyefoods?
People of all ages will benefit from adding eyefoods to their diets. Eyefoods contain nutrients that help prevent the progression of an existing eye condition and reduce the risk of developing eye disease and experiencing vision loss.

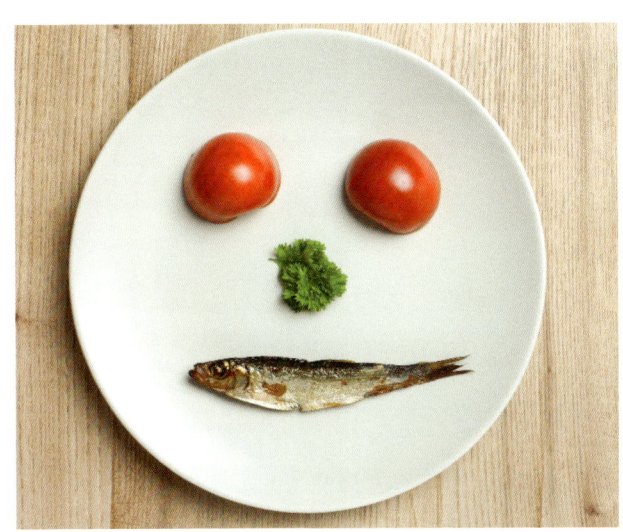

Introduction

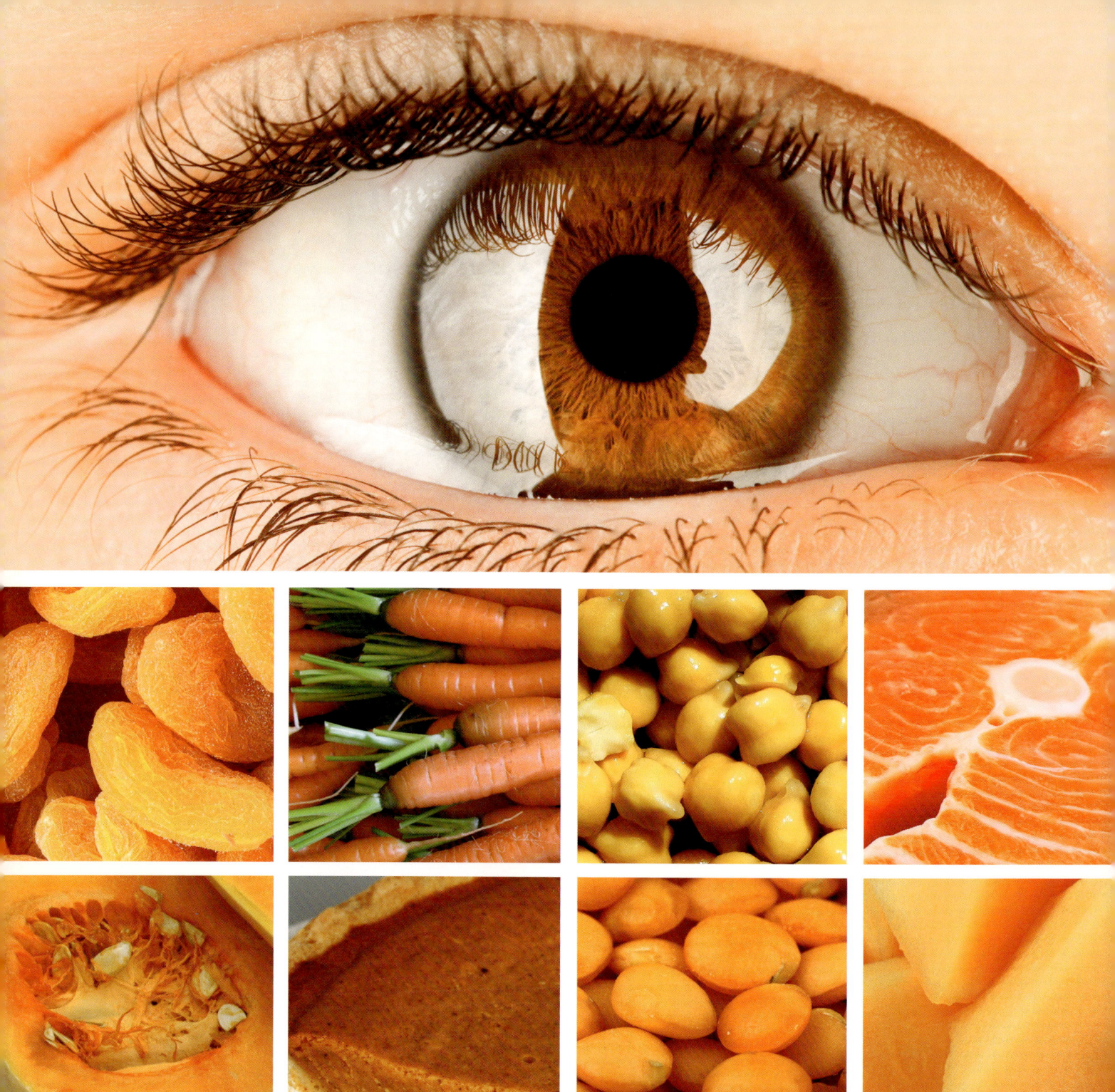

Part One
The Basics

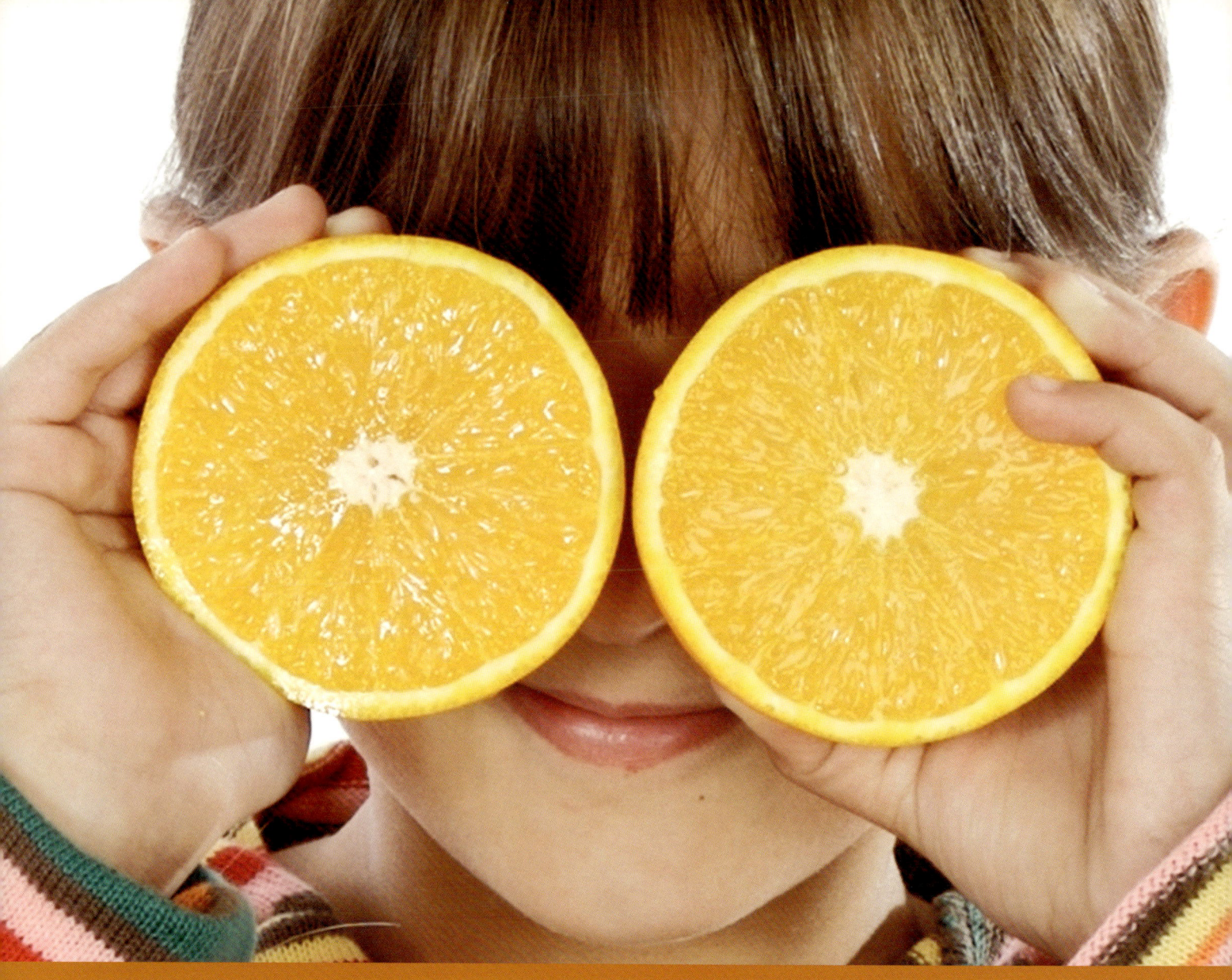

The first step in the prevention of eye disease is awareness. Many common eye diseases are strongly linked to diet, environment, and lifestyle.

Chapter 1
Eye Health and Disease

During our years of optometric practice, we have found that most people consider vision to be one of their most important senses. Maintaining healthy eyes is a priority to everyone, and our patients frequently ask how they can keep their eyes strong and preserve their vision. Current research has taught us that the risk of many eye diseases can be decreased with a proper diet and lifestyle. You hold the keys to your eye health.

Learning about eye health and eye disease is the first step in preserving vision or dealing with an existing eye condition. Many people wear glasses or contact lenses to see better at a distance, for reading, or for both. Most people who wear glasses or contact lenses do not have eye disease, but rather an eye condition called *refractive error*, more commonly known as nearsightedness (myopia), farsightedness (hyperopia), astigmatism, or prespbyopia (loss of focusing ability).

This chapter describes the most common eye diseases, including their symptoms, causes, and treatments. It is not a comprehensive list of all eye diseases, but focuses on chronic eye conditions, most of which are related to aging or inflammation in the body. These are the diseases that are most likely to be influenced by diet.

Remember, though, that each person is different, and eye disease can present differently in everyone. If you do think you might suffer from an eye condition, speak with your eye doctor.

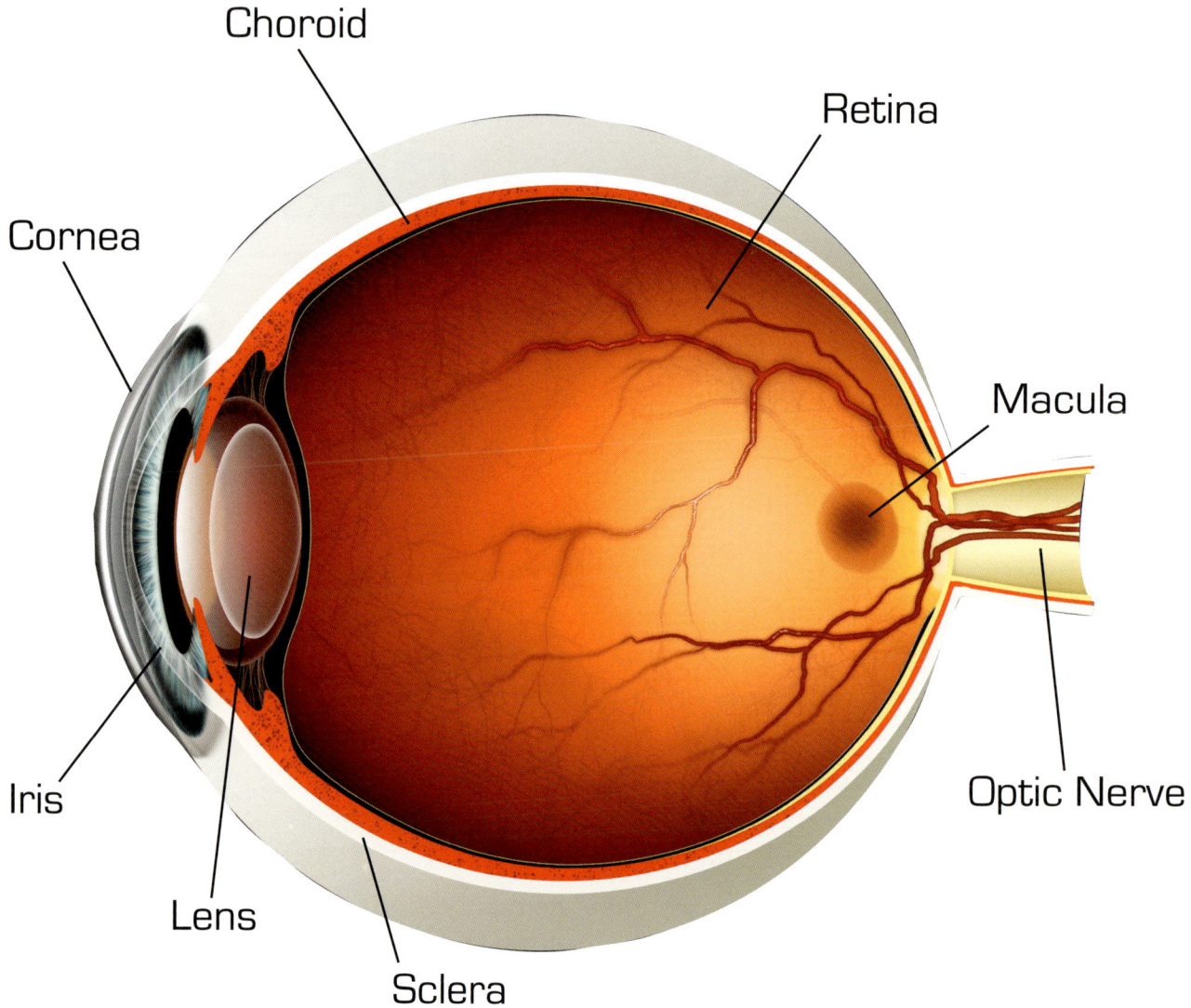

The Canadian Association of Optometrists recommends the following guidelines for eye examinations for people who are at low risk for developing eye problems.

Age Group	Minimum recommended frequency of eye examination
Infants and toddlers (Birth to 24 months)	By age six months
Preschool children (2-5 years)	At age three and before entering elementary school
School age (6-19 years)	Annually
Adult (20-64 years)	Every one to two years
Older adult (65 years and older)	Annually

Information in the table retrieved from the Canadian Association of Optometrists website. www.opto.ca/en/optometry/exam-frequency.html (July 2010)

Eye Health and Disease   Chapter 1

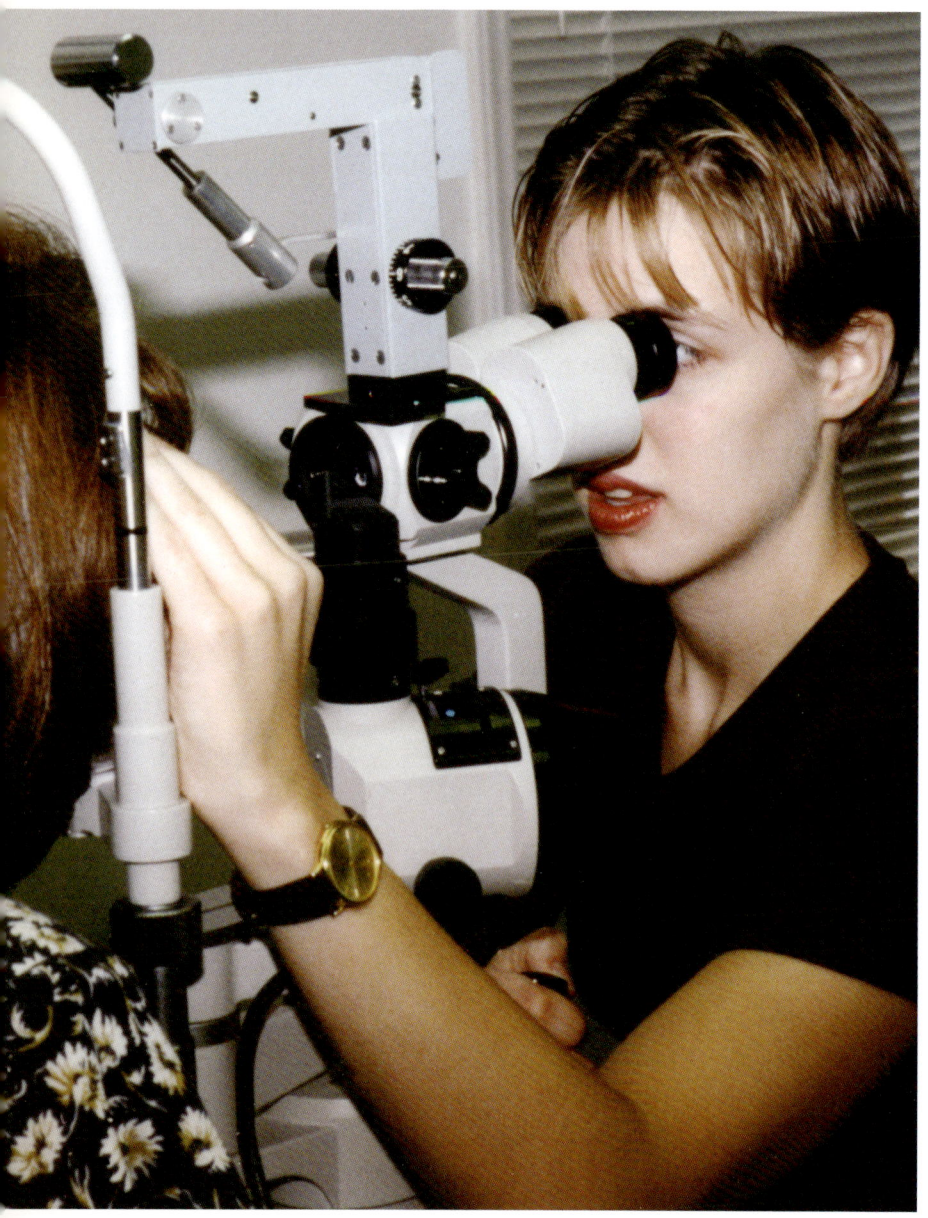

Regular eye examinations by an optometrist or ophthalmologist are important for early diagnosis and treatment of eye conditions. Even if you have never had any vision problems, regular eye examinations will help prevent vision loss from eye disease. An optometrist or ophthalmologist can diagnose many eye diseases that do not have noticeable symptoms.

- After your first comprehensive eye examination, your eye doctor will determine if more frequent eye exams are necessary.

Part 1   The Basics

Common Eye Diseases

Age-Related Macular Degeneration (AMD)

What is Age-related macular degeneration (AMD)?

Age-related macular degeneration (AMD) is a chronic disease of the central part of the retina, the macula. It is the leading cause of blindness in the Western world. Researchers estimate that over 2 million Canadians have some form of AMD. As the population ages, this number is expected to increase significantly. Currently, the Eye Disease Prevalence research group estimates that 1.8 million Americans have advanced AMD, and that this number is likely to double in the next two decades.[3]

There are two forms of AMD: dry AMD and wet AMD. Dry AMD is more common than wet AMD. Dry AMD can lead to wet AMD.

Dry AMD: Dry AMD occurs when cells in the macula begin to break down, causing thinning of the macula and a gradual decrease in vision. In addition, the retina becomes unable to rid itself of its metabolic waste, called lipofuscin. Lipofuscin accumulates in the retina as drusen, which block the normal function of the retina.

Wet AMD: Wet AMD is caused by the growth of abnormal blood vessels in the choroid, which provides the blood supply of the retina. These new blood vessels grow into the macula through breaks in the membrane that separates the choroid from the retina. These weak blood vessels leak fluid into the retina, leading to a decrease in vision that is more rapid and dramatic than in dry AMD.

Neither dry AMD nor wet AMD causes total blindness, only a decrease or loss of central vision. People with AMD may notice changes in their ability to read books, to see street signs, or to see details on a person's face; however, they are able to walk and move around safely.

Eye Health and Disease   Chapter 1

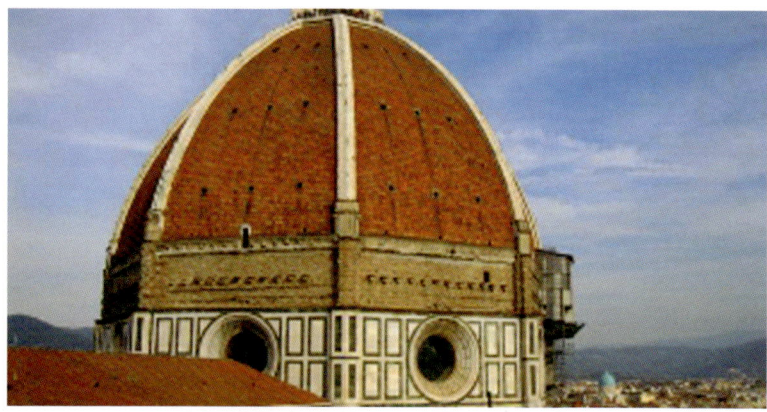

Normal vision.

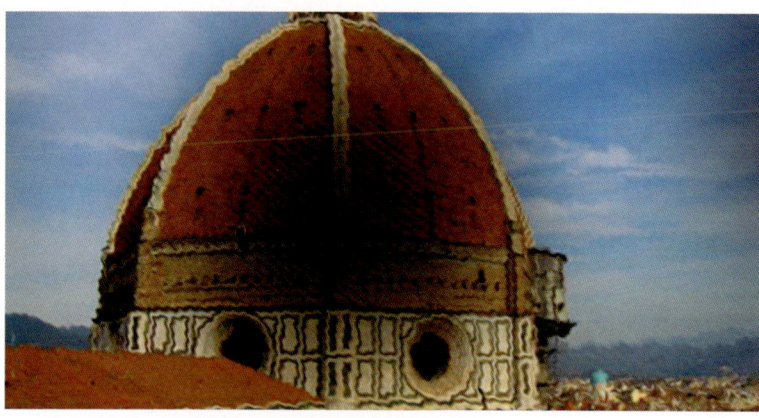

An example of the vision of a person with early AMD.

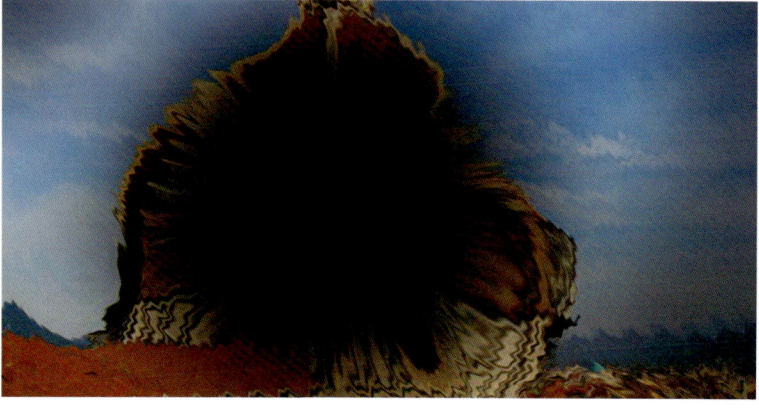

An example of the vision of a person with advanced AMD

Part 1   The Basics

What are the symptoms of AMD?
- Gradual loss of central vision
- Distortion of straight lines
- Blurry vision when reading
- Rapid-onset loss of central vision
- Blind spot in or near the central vision
- AMD can also be asymptomatic

What are the risk factors for AMD?
- Age
- Smoking
- Family history of AMD
- UV light exposure
- Blue light exposure (short wavelength visible light)
- Diets high in sugar and refined carbohydrates
- Excess weight or obesity
- Gender (women are at a higher risk than men)
- Eye color (light colored eyes have a higher risk)
- Race (Caucasians are at a higher risk)
- Diabetes
- Cardiovascular disease

How is AMD diagnosed?
An optometrist or ophthalmologist can diagnose AMD during a dilated eye examination using special lenses. Other tests that aid in the diagnosis of AMD include a thorough patient history, Amsler grid testing, and advanced imaging of the retina with specialized equipment. An optometrist or ophthalmologist will often diagnose early AMD during a routine eye examination, before a person has any symptoms. Early diagnosis of AMD can give a person the opportunity to make diet and lifestyle changes that decrease the risk of progression of the disease.

Controlling AMD with diet:
Numerous studies have shown a relationship between nutrition and AMD. To date, the most significant study in the field of AMD and nutrition is the Age-Related Eye Disease Study (AREDS). AREDS was a large randomized controlled trial that followed over 3,000 participants for seven years and concluded that taking a supplement with specific antioxidants and zinc decreases the risk of progression of AMD in certain patients by as much as 25%.[4]

Eye Health and Disease   Chapter 1

The follow-up study, AREDS-2, is currently assessing the preventative effects of supplementing patients' diets with high doses of two carotenoids (lutein and zeaxanthin) and omega-3 fatty acids.

Eyecare professionals recommend that most patients with AMD take an AREDS-type vitamin supplement and an omega-3 fatty acid supplement. However, a supplement is not a replacement for a healthy diet. The synergy of the nutrients in whole foods has a beneficial effect on our bodies that a supplement cannot replicate. Many other studies have found that diets high in certain nutrients help to reduce the risk of AMD, and that poor diets can increase a person's risk for developing the disease. The findings of these studies are summarized in the lists below:

Prevention of AMD through diet[5]:
- Eat foods rich in the carotenoids lutein and zeaxanthin
- Ensure your diet is high in vitamin C, vitamin E, beta-carotene and zinc
- Choose fish with high levels of omega-3 fatty acids
- Engage in a higher level of physical activity or exercise

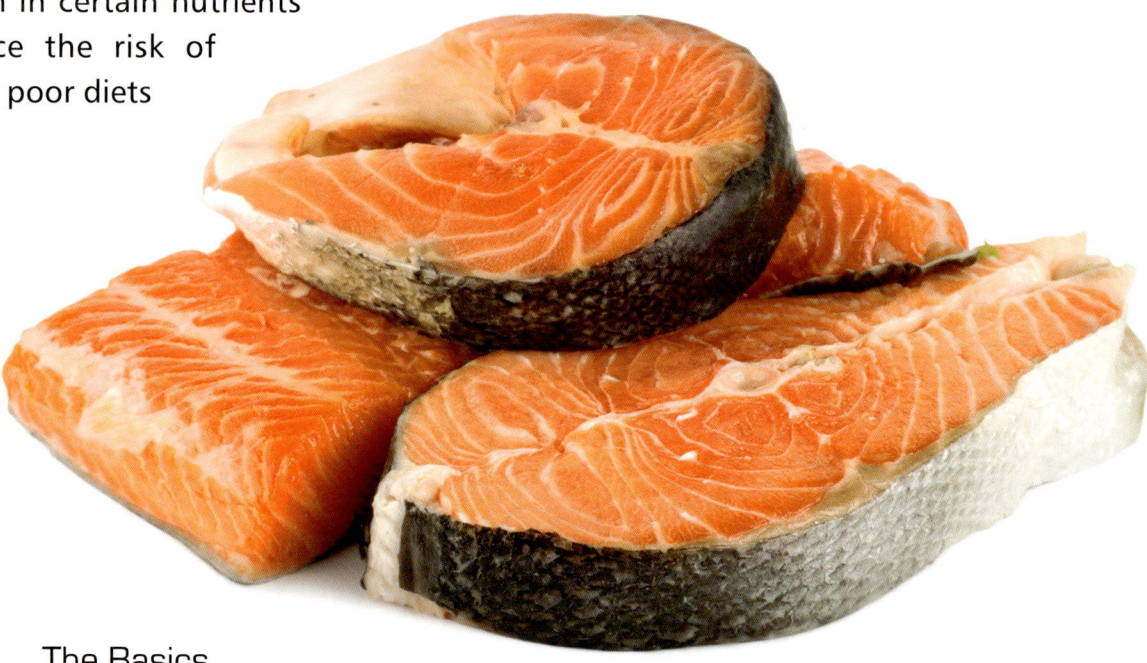

Part 1   The Basics

Risk factors[6]:
- A diet with a high glycemic index
- Excess weight and obesity

The field of research for treatments for dry and wet AMD is constantly evolving. Even at the writing of this book, the treatment options for the disease are changing and improving.

What is the current treatment for dry AMD?

The current treatment for dry AMD aims to slow the progression of the disease. If you have dry AMD, you are advised to modify your diet and lifestyle by eating foods rich in specific antioxidants and omega-3 fatty acids, to take AREDS-based ocular vitamins, to wear sunglasses, and to stop smoking. Optometrists and ophthalmologists advise people with dry AMD to use an Amsler grid on a daily basis. The Amsler grid is a simple test that allows a person to notice subtle changes in vision that can be a sign of progression of dry AMD to wet AMD.

What is the current treatment for wet AMD?

There are several treatment options for wet AMD, depending on the stage of the disease and the location of the abnormal blood vessels. These include laser photocoagulation, photodynamic therapy with Visudyne®, and anti-VEGF (vaso-endothelial growth factor) injections. To date, the only treatment that has shown an improvement in visual acuity is anti-VEGF medication.

Anti-VEGF medications block the protein (VEGF) that is responsible for new blood vessel growth. In wet AMD, these medications help stop the growth of new blood vessels in the retina. They may slow the progression of vision loss and, in some cases, even improve vision. An ophthalmologist will inject the medication into the eye. Multiple injections, given on a monthly basis, are often required for the treatment to be effective.[7]

Age-Related Macular Degeneration (AMD)

IN SUMMARY

- AMD is the leading cause of blindness in the Western world.
- AMD affects central vision only. It does not lead to total blindness.
- There are two types of AMD: dry AMD and wet AMD.
- Dry AMD is more common and less severe than wet AMD. In some cases, dry AMD can progress to wet AMD.
- Antioxidants, carotenoids (lutein and zeaxanthin), omega-3 fatty acids, and diets high in fiber that include whole grains may help to prevent or reduce the risk of progression of AMD.
- People with signs of early to intermediate AMD are generally advised by their optometrist or ophthalmologist to take an AREDS-based vitamin supplement, to follow a diet filled with eyefoods, and to visit their eye doctor regularly.
- Smoking increases the risk of AMD.[8]

Part 1   The Basics

Cataracts

What are cataracts?
A cataract is a condition in which the lens of the eye loses its transparency. As we age, the lenses in our eyes become cloudy, causing a gradual blurring of vision along with reduced night vision. Many people are not aware that they have cataracts because the change in their vision is so gradual.

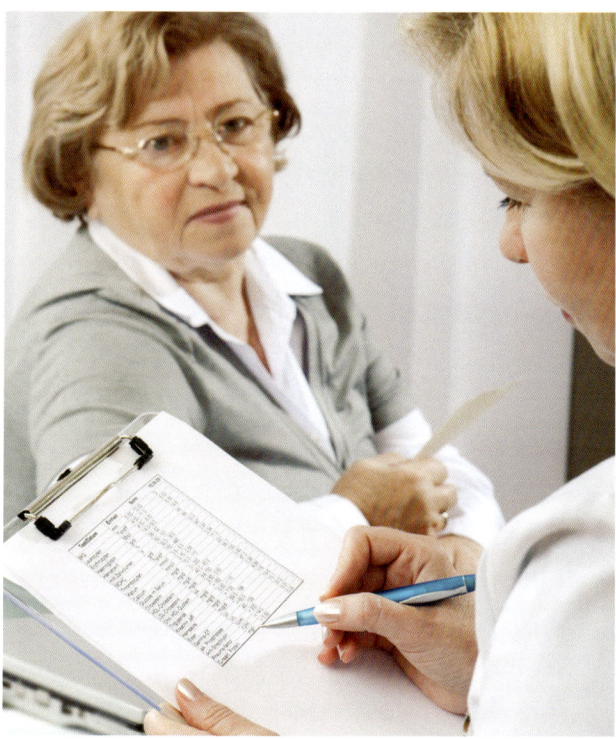

Cataracts are most common in people over the age of 60; however, certain types of cataracts can occur in younger people. There are three main types of cataracts: nuclear sclerosis, anterior cortical cataract, and posterior subcapsular cataract. In most cases, a cataract presents itself as a combination of the three types.

What are the symptoms of cataracts?
- Reduced distance–and/or near vision
- Dim or blurry vision
- Difficulty driving at night
- Glare
- More light required for reading
- Increased nearsightedness

What are the risk factors for cataracts?
- Age
- Medications (steroids taken over long periods of time increase the risk of posterior subcapsular cataracts)
- UV light exposure
- Family history (helps to predict when cataracts will develop)
- Diets excessively high in sugar and refined carbohydrates[9]

Eye Health and Disease   Chapter 1

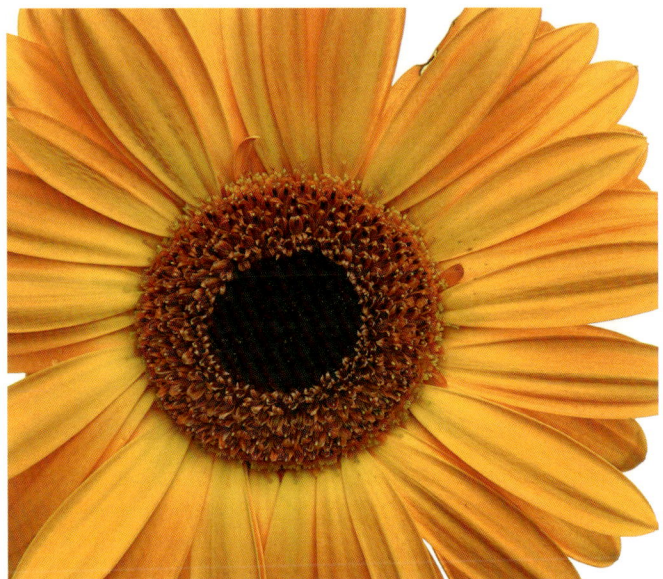

The image below is an example of the vision of a person with cataracts.

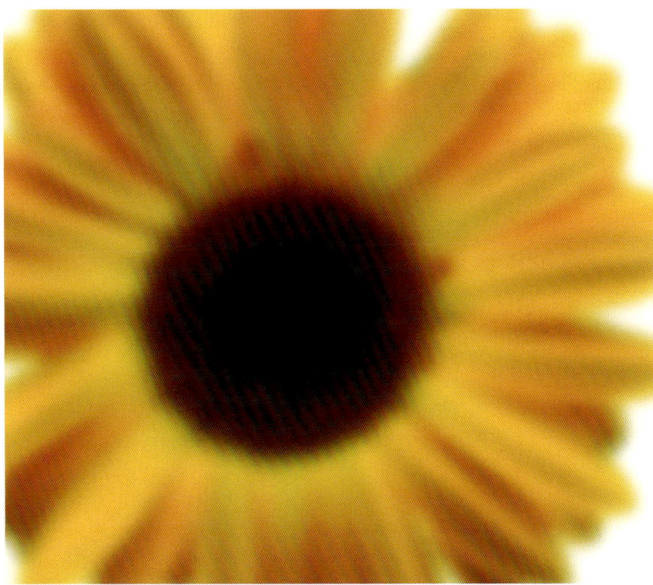

How are cataracts diagnosed?
An optometrist or ophthalmologist can diagnose cataracts by using a high-powered microscope during a dilated eye examination.

Controlling cataracts with diet[10]:
- Diets rich in antioxidants and the carotenoids lutein and zeaxanthin may offer protection against the development of cataracts.
- Diets consisting of foods with a high glycemic index may increase the risk for cataracts.
- Diets high in omega-3 fatty acids may decrease the risk of certain types of cataracts.

What is the current treatment for cataracts?
Cataracts progress at different rates in different people, so if you have cataracts it is important to talk to your eye doctor about the stage of your cataracts. If you have early signs of cataracts, you may be able to delay their progression by

Part 1   The Basics

consuming a diet rich in foods that promote eye health (eyefoods) and by wearing sunglasses to protect your eyes from UV and blue light.

Cataract surgery is the only treatment for advanced cataracts. An ophthalmologist performs cataract surgery on patients if the cataracts are visually and clinically significant.

If cataract surgery is required, the surgeon will use an ultrasound technology (phaco-emulsification) to break up the cataract before it is removed. The surgeon then removes the lens of the eye and replaces it with an intraocular lens implant. Many different types of intraocular lens implants are available, so remember to ask your eye surgeon which intraocular lens implant will be best for you.

Cataract surgery is generally a safe procedure and the risk for complications in cataract surgery is very low. Most people feel no pain or discomfort during or after surgery. The surgery is performed in either a hospital or a clinic, depending on regional policies.

Healing and recovery time after cataract surgery will vary, though many people see an improvement in their vision within a few days. Most people will no longer require glasses for seeing at a distance, though they may still have to use reading glasses. Your surgeon or optometrist will assess your eyes at scheduled follow-up visits.

Cataracts

IN SUMMARY

- A cataract is a loss of transparency in the lens of the eye.
- Cataracts are most commonly seen in people over the age of 60.
- Cataracts usually progress slowly, causing a gradual change in vision.
- Antioxidants, carotenoids (lutein and zeaxanthin) and omega-3 fatty acids may protect against the development or progression of cataracts.
- Diets with a high glycemic index have been shown to increase the risk of cataracts.
- UV light exposure increases the risk of cataracts.
- Cataract surgery, a low-risk procedure with a high success rate, is the only treatment for cataracts.
- During cataract surgery, a surgeon implants an intraocular lens into the eye, often eliminating the need for glasses for seeing in the distance.

Dry Eye Syndrome

What is dry eye syndrome?
Dry eye syndrome is a very common eye condition that affects men and women of all ages. Even though it usually does not cause significant vision loss like AMD or cataracts, dry eye syndrome does have a significant impact on overall eye health, and the symptoms can affect a person's quality of life. Dry eye syndrome is often called *ocular surface disease*. It does not necessarily mean that a person has a deficiency of tears but an imbalance of the tear film.

The tear film is composed of three layers: aqueous (water), lipid (oil), and mucous. In dry eye syndrome, various factors disrupt the balance of these three layers.

The symptoms of dry eye syndrome vary greatly. People who suffer from this condition rarely report that their eyes actually feel dry. Dry eye syndrome affects people of all ages with varying degrees of severity. Mild dry eye syndrome may cause the feeling that something is in the eye or a burning sensation. Moderate to severe dry eye syndrome can cause eye pain and profound watering of the eyes.

What are the symptoms of dry eye syndrome?
- Burning eyes
- Watery eyes
- Foreign-body sensation
- Redness
- Discharge
- Light sensitivity

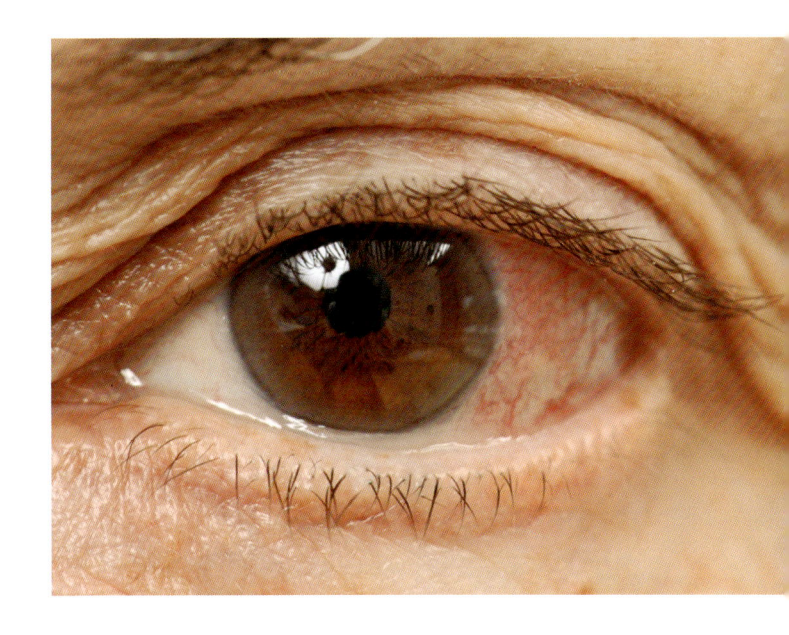

Eye Health and Disease   Chapter 1

What are the causes of dry eye syndrome?
- Environment
- Eyelid disease (blepharitis or meibomianitis)
- Dietary imbalance (High omega-6 : omega-3 intake ratio)
- Medication
- Systemic disease (such as Sjogren's syndrome or rheumatoid arthritis)
- Contact lenses
- Computer use

How is dry eye syndrome diagnosed?

An optometrist or ophthalmologist will diagnose dry eye syndrome using a variety of tests. In most cases, your eye doctor can diagnose dry eye syndrome by looking at your eyes with a high-powered microscope. A detailed patient history, including a description of the symptoms and their duration, is important in the diagnosis of dry eye syndrome. Other tests used to diagnose this condition are the Schirmer tear test and an assessment of the cornea using specialized eye drops.

Controlling dry eye syndrome with diet[11]:
- Omega-3 fatty acids can decrease the incidence of dry eye syndrome in women. Indeed, an in-depth study showed that women with a higher dietary intake of omega-3 fatty acids (mainly from cold water fish such as tuna) have a lower prevalence of dry eye syndrome.
- Diets with a high omega-6 to omega-3 ratio (15:1) are associated with an incidence of dry eye syndrome that is twice as high as that seen in diets with a low ratio.
- Flax seed oil can improve the symptoms of dry eye syndrome in patients with Sjogren's syndrome (a disease characterized by dry mucous membranes in the body).

What is the treatment for dry eye syndrome?

There are many treatment options available for dry eye syndrome, depending on the cause and severity of the condition. The most important factor in the success of dry

With patience and perseverance, some of the following treatments can decrease the symptoms of dry eye syndrome.

- Artificial tear drops
- Warm compresses and eyelid scrubs (a special product to cleanse the eyelids)
- Anti-inflammatory medications (such as Restasis® or mild steroid eye drops)
- Omega-3 fatty acids (preferably from cold water fish sources)
- Punctal occlusion (blocking tear ducts to decrease tear drainage)

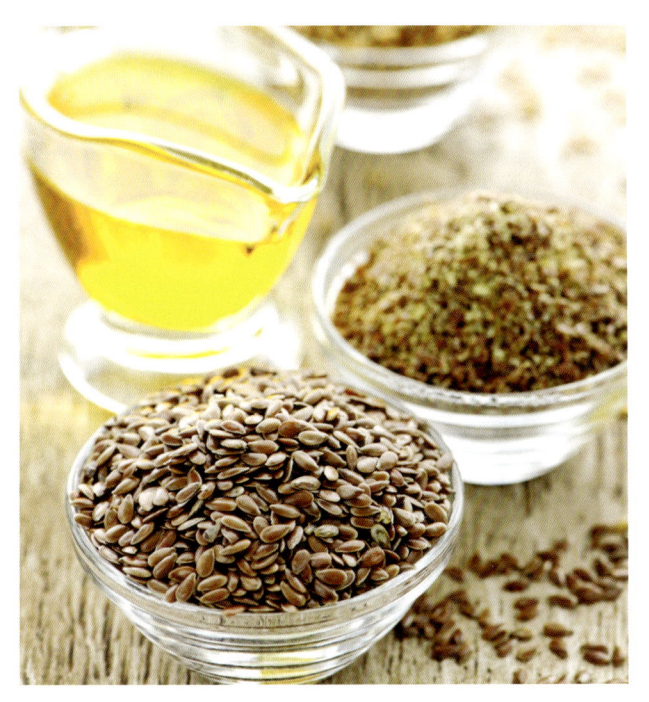

eye treatment is patient compliance. Many people find the treatment too much trouble and do not follow through with their doctors' recommendations. This can lead to frustration and discouragement for both the patient and the doctor.

If you think you may have dry eye syndrome, discuss your treatment options with your eye doctor. Be aware that the treatment of your condition will be an involved process and may require frequent follow-up visits.

In our optometric practices, we see patients every day who are suffering from dry eye syndrome. Most people are looking for a quick cure for their symptoms. However, what they do not realize is that dry eye syndrome is a chronic disease, and that the symptoms are a sign of inflammation in the eye. Just as it takes time for dry eye syndrome to cause discomfort, burning, or watering of the eyes, so does the treatment take time to be effective.

Eye Health and Disease   Chapter 1

Dry Eye Syndrome

IN SUMMARY

- Dry eye syndrome is a common chronic eye condition that affects people of all ages with varying degrees of severity.
- Dry eye syndrome does not cause vision loss, but it can cause fluctuating vision, making reading more difficult. Untreated moderate to severe dry eye syndrome can affect a person's quality of life.
- The symptoms vary depending on the cause of dry eye syndrome and the severity.
- Often people with dry eye syndrome will experience watering of their eyes.
- Environmental factors can affect the severity of the symptoms of dry eye syndrome.
- Omega-3 fatty acids from fish and flax seed oil can help relieve dry eye syndrome in certain people.
- Patience is required in the treatment of dry eye syndrome. With proper care and diet adjustments, the symptoms can be greatly reduced.

Eyelid Disorders

Blepharitis and meibomianitis

Blepharitis and meibomianitis are common chronic disorders of the eyelid that are often associated with dry eye syndrome. Blepharitis is an inflammation of the eyelid margin. Meibomianitis is inflammation of the oil glands in the eyelid. Blepharitis and meibomianitis usually occur together. They are chronic conditions for which there is no cure. However, ongoing treatment can minimize the signs and symptoms of blepharitis and meibomianitis.

In people with eyelid disorders, the oil glands in the eyelids do not function properly. As a result, the eyelids become inflamed and the normal bacteria that reside on the eyelashes proliferate. If left untreated, severe eyelid disorders can lead to the development of styes, chalazia (chronic styes), or corneal ulcers caused by sensitivity to the staphylococcal bacteria found on the eyelid.

What are the symptoms of eyelid disorders?
- Eyelid redness
- Burning
- Discomfort
- Foreign-body sensation
- Watery eyes
- Discharge (mucous or sleep in the eyes, especially in the morning)

What are the causes of eyelid disorders?
- Acne rosacea
- Dietary imbalance
- Inflammation
- Environment
- Idiopathic (unknown cause)

How are eyelid disorders diagnosed?
An optometrist or ophthalmologist can diagnose eyelid disorders during an eye examination by using a high-powered microscope. A detailed history of your ocular symptoms also aids in the diagnosis of eyelid disorders.

Controlling eyelid disorders with diet:
An imbalance of fatty acids in the body

Eye Health and Disease   Chapter 1

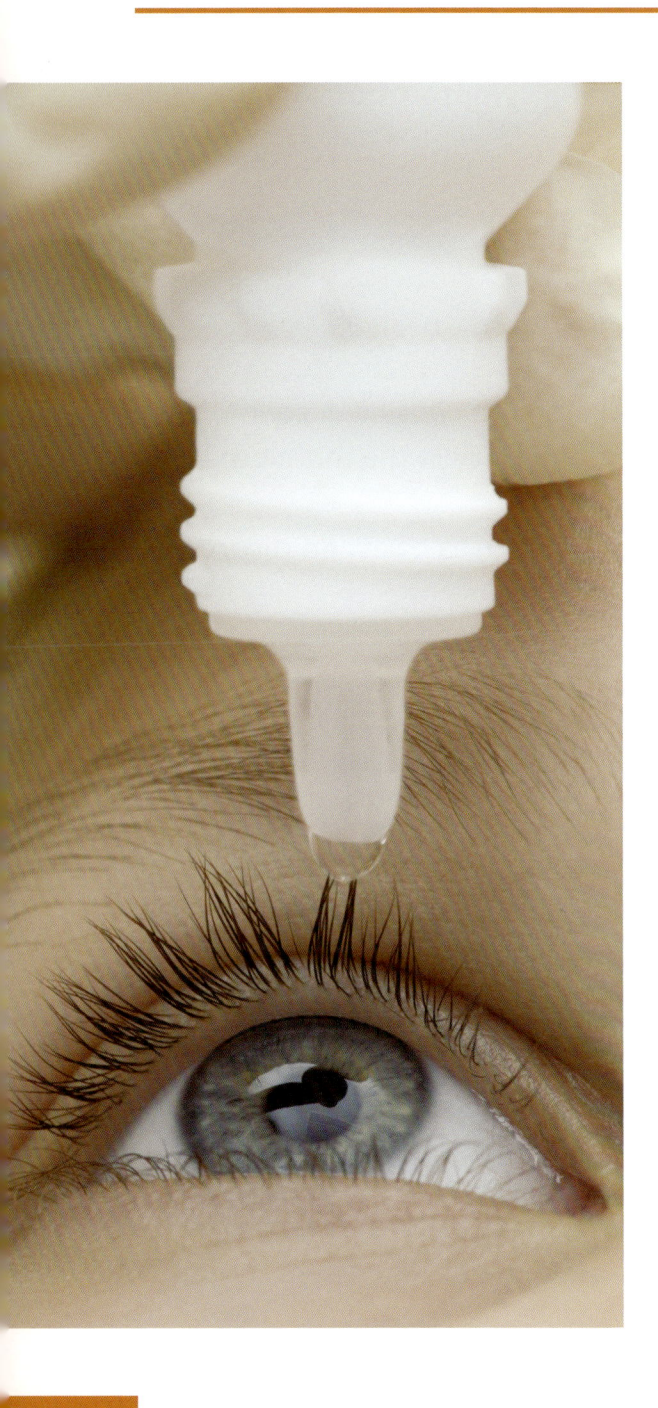

promotes inflammation in the body. The typical North American diet does not include enough omega-3 fatty acids. As a result, inflammatory conditions such as blepharitis and meibomianitis are common in North America. People with skin conditions such as acne rosacea are also prone to developing eyelid disorders.[12]

What is the treatment for blepharitis and meibomianitis?

There are different courses of treatment for blepharitis and meibomianitis, depending on the severity and type of eyelid disorder. Most treatment regimens include applying warm compresses to the upper and lower eyelids for up to five minutes at least once a day. This treatment is followed by eyelid hygiene that involves using a special product to cleanse the eyelid margins. These procedures help to control the build-up of oils and bacteria at the eyelid margins.

- Warm compresses to the eyelids
- Eyelid hygiene
- Artificial tears
- Omega-3 fatty acids in diet

Part 1   The Basics

- Anti-inflammatory eye drops or combination anti-inflammatory–antibiotic eye drops (short term therapy)
- Oral antibiotics (used for their anti-inflammatory properties)

As with dry eye syndrome, blepharitis and meibomianitis are chronic conditions for which there is no cure. Remember that the symptoms of eyelid disorders only occur after there is inflammation. Therefore, treatment for eyelid disorders takes time. Once the symptoms have lessened and your eyes feel better, it is important to continue the treatment regimen. Maintaining healthy eyes takes commitment. If you currently have an eyelid disorder, just a few changes to your daily routine and diet will lead to healthy eyes.

Inflammation in the Body

In many cases, inflammation is important to our health. It occurs as the body's natural response to injury or to foreign invaders such as bacteria or viruses. Inflammation is the cornerstone of healing. However, inflammation can also occur for no beneficial reason to the body. This is the case in autoimmune diseases such as rheumatoid arthritis, lupus, and ankylosing spondylitis.

The symptoms of dry eye syndrome, blepharitis, and meibomianitis are the result of inflammation in the eye. Without treatment, these conditions cause inflammation to occur on the surface of the eye.

Many factors in the North American lifestyle lead to chronic inflammation in the body. Smoking, obesity, and an imbalance in dietary intake of omega-6 and omega-3 fatty acids (i.e. 15:1) are all considered to be pro-inflammatory. Chronic inflammation is a risk factor in diseases such as atherosclerosis, type 2 diabetes, and even cancer.[13]

Eye Health and Disease   Chapter 1

Eyelid Disorders

IN SUMMARY

- Blepharitis and meibomianitis are common eyelid disorders that are chronic in nature.
- There is no cure for blepharitis and meibomianitis, but daily treatment routines can minimize or eliminate the symptoms of these conditions.
- Though there are many causes for eyelid disorders, the underlying cause is inflammation.
- The anti-inflammatory properties of omega-3 fatty acids may help blepharitis and meibomianitis by decreasing inflammation.
- Successful treatment of blepharitis and meibomianitis requires daily routines as recommended by an optometrist or ophthalmologist.
- Routine follow-up appointments are important in the treatment of eyelid disorders. In certain cases, oral medications may be necessary.
- Be patient. With proper treatment, the symptoms of eyelid disorders can improve greatly.

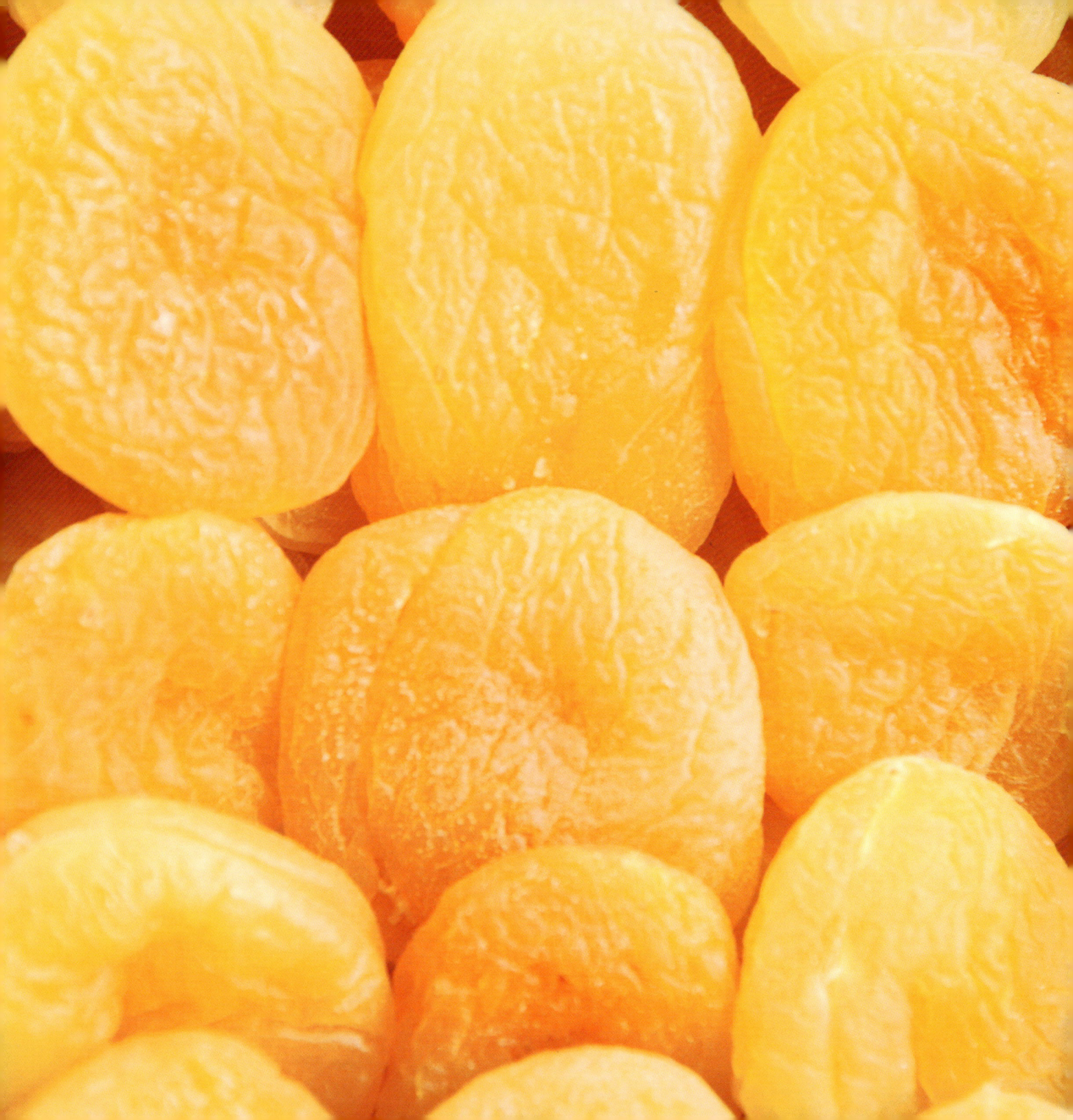

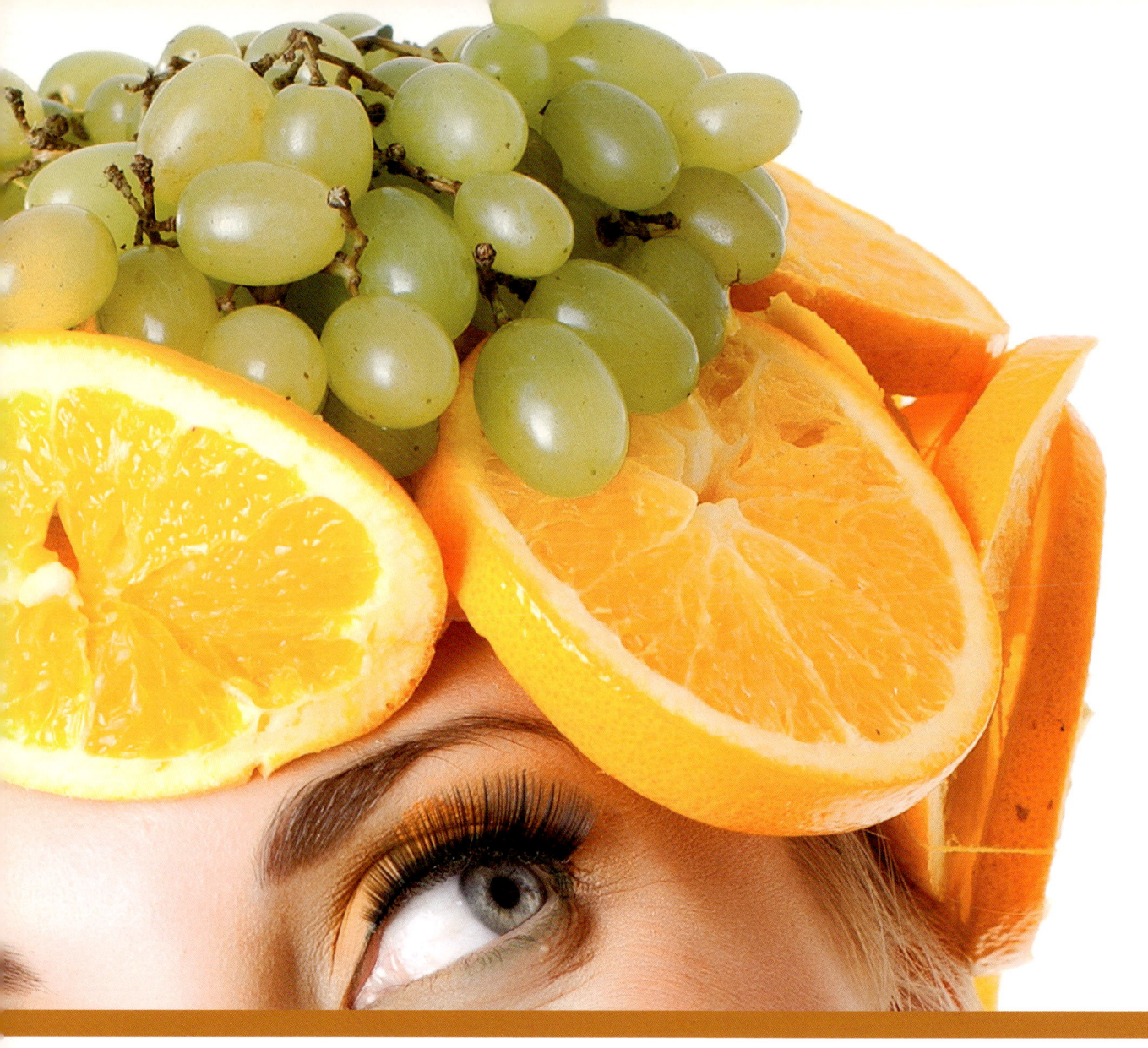

After careful review of scientific studies, we have determined the most important nutrients for the prevention of eye disease and the promotion of eye health. Eyefoods are full of the nutrients that are essential for eye health.

Chapter 2
Eye Nutrients

Eye nutrients are a group of nutrients that are beneficial to eye health. After careful review of scientific studies, we have determined the most important nutrients for the prevention of eye disease and the promotion of eye health. Each of these nutrients may decrease the risk of eye disease, either on its own or in conjunction with other nutrients. In addition to these nutrients, we focus on dietary factors such as glycemic index and fiber intake.

In our optometric practice, we encounter questions from our patients on the use of vitamins, minerals, and supplements to promote eye health. Most people have heard that antioxidants are important for healthy eyes. Some are aware of the importance of specific nutrients such as lutein and zeaxanthin to the eyes. However, the majority of people have questions about how to use this information and how to add these nutrients to their diets.

In this chapter, we will describe the most important eye nutrients. Even though the nutrients may help to prevent eye disease on their own, it is the synergy of nutrients that best maintains eye health. The Eyefoods and Eyefoods Plan chapters will show you how to benefit from this nutrient synergy.

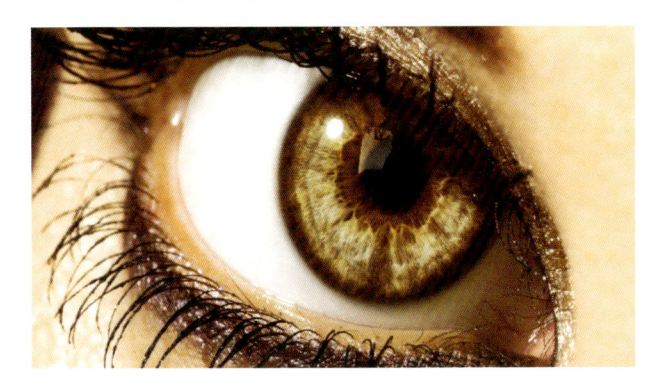

Eye Nutrients   Chapter 2

Frequently Asked Nutrition Questions

Should I take vitamin supplements, or is it better to try to achieve an adequate nutrient intake from my diet?
People with certain ocular and medical conditions or risk factors for certain diseases will not be able to meet the nutritional requirements necessary for disease prevention through diet alone. In these cases, it is important to take a supplement if advised by a health care professional. However, a supplement is not a replacement for a healthy diet. The synergy of nutrients in whole foods has beneficial effects on our bodies that supplements cannot replicate.

As mentioned in Chapter 1, eye care professionals will advise most people with early age-related macular degeneration (AMD) to take an AREDS-type vitamin supplement and an omega-3 fatty acid supplement to help prevent the progression of AMD. In the following chapter, we will review the benefits that certain nutrients have on eye health and general health as shown in scientific studies.

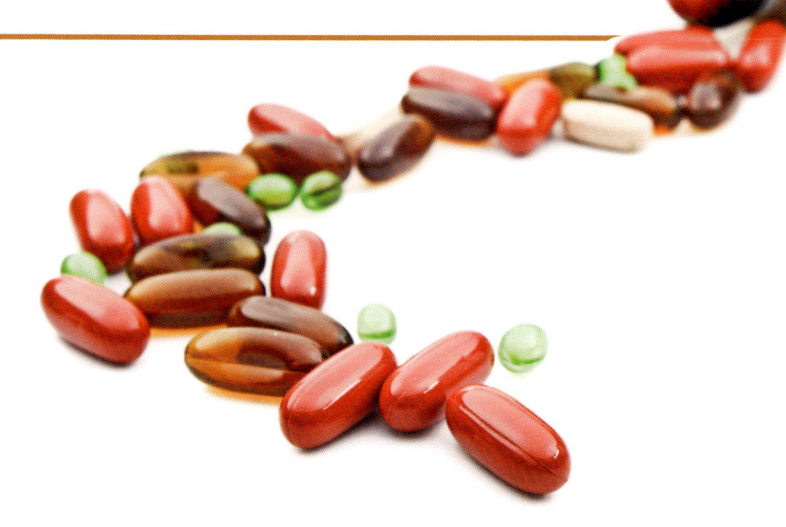

You should make the decision to take a supplement only after you have had a discussion with your health care provider. Pregnant women, breastfeeding women, and people with health conditions need to check with a physician before taking a supplement. Some supplements can interact with certain prescription and over-the-counter medications, causing adverse side effects or altering the efficacy of the medication. For this reason, it is important to inform your health care providers of all the prescription and non-prescription drugs or supplements you are taking.

Part 1   The Basics

How much of each nutrient do I need?
The recommended dosage of each nutrient varies for people with different medical conditions and for healthy individuals. For disease prevention or management, your health care professional will follow the guidelines of current scientific research to determine the appropriate amount of each nutrient for you. For healthy individuals, the Institute of Medicine (a department of the United States National Institute of Health) has issued reference values for nutrient intakes called Dietary Reference Intakes (DRI). Health Canada uses the DRI to determine adequate nutrient intakes for healthy population groups that are not at high risk for disease. Sometimes, specific scientific studies will be published that recommend doses of nutrients higher than those in the DRI. These conflicting reports can cause confusion, so it is always important to discuss this with your health care provider.

There are four values as part of the DRI.[14] In this chapter, we will refer to the following three DRI values for eye nutrients.

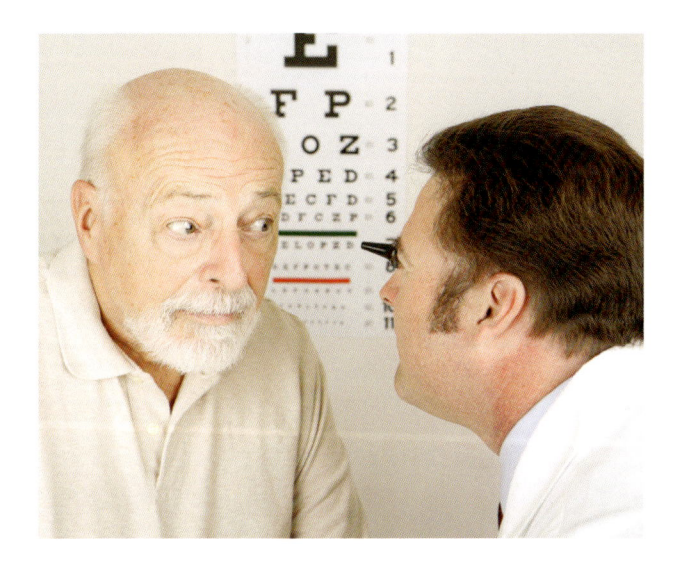

RDA (recommended dietary allowance): The average daily intake of a nutrient that is enough to meet the dietary requirements for healthy individuals. The RDA changes according to age group and gender.

AI (adequate intake): The estimated average intake of a nutrient for a healthy population. It is applicable when an RDA cannot be determined.

UL (tolerable upper intake level): The highest usual daily intake of a nutrient that is likely to have no adverse effects. The UL is dependent on gender and age group.

Eye Nutrients   Chapter 2

An Overview of Eye Nutrients

Nutrient	Description	Common Food Sources
Lutein & Zeaxanthin	Carotenoid	Fruits and vegetables, eggs
Omega-3 Fatty Acids	DHA, EPA, ALA	Cold water fish, some plant oils
Vitamin C	Antioxidant	Fruits and vegetables
Beta-Carotene	Carotenoid	Fruits and vegetables
Vitamin E	Antioxidant	Oils, nuts, eggs, some fruits and vegetables
Zinc	Essential mineral	Seafood, meat, nuts, whole grains, fortified breakfast cereals
Fiber	Plant compounds	Whole grains, fruits and vegetables

Part 1   The Basics

Antioxidants

Antioxidants are a class of substances that help to prevent oxidation in the body. They include vitamins and minerals such as vitamin C, vitamin E, and selenium, as well as phytochemicals such as the carotenoids lutein and zeaxanthin.

What is oxidation?
Oxidation is a chemical reaction within the body that changes a stable molecule into a free radical. Exposure to certain environmental factors, including UV light, hazardous chemicals, and air pollution, causes free radicals to form. The natural aging process, poor dietary habits, and smoking also trigger their formation. If left unchecked, free radicals will damage body tissues and can lead to a variety of chronic and age-related diseases such as AMD, cancer, and cardiovascular disease.

What are carotenoids?
Carotenoids are a group of over 600 naturally occurring pigments. Of all carotenoids, the most important to our bodies are beta-carotene, lutein, zeaxanthin, lycopene, alpha-carotene, and beta-cryptoxanthin. Carotenoids give fruits and vegetables their bright colors.

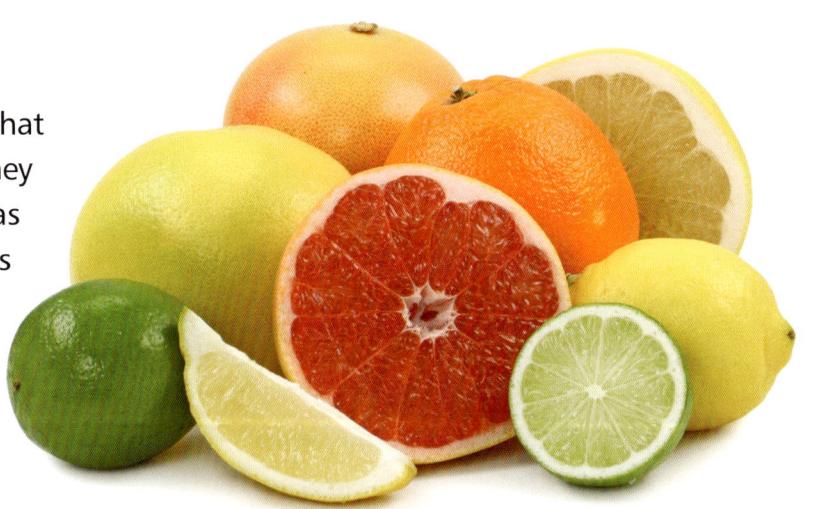

Antioxidants and eye disease:
Antioxidants may reduce the risk of age-related macular degeneration and cataracts.[15]

Antioxidants and general health:
Antioxidants have been shown to reduce the risk of cardiovascular disease, respiratory disease, and cancer. They can also enhance immune function.[16]

Lutein and Zeaxanthin

Lutein and zeaxanthin are pigments that are abundant in the macula (the central part of the retina). Our bodies cannot make lutein and zeaxanthin; therefore, we must obtain them from our diet. In the eye, lutein and zeaxanthin absorb blue-and UV light, protecting the macula from their harmful effects. Consuming lutein and zeaxanthin, either in foods or in a supplement, results in an increase of carotenoids in the macula.

Lutein and zeaxanthin are abundant in fruits and vegetables. Lutein is found in leafy green vegetables and egg yolks; zeaxanthin in orange peppers.[17] Adding oil to foods high in lutein will significantly increase your body's absorption of lutein.[18]

Dietary Reference Intakes

RDA: To date no RDA has been set. The Institute of Medicine recommends consumption of carotenoid-rich fruits and vegetables.

UL: To date no UL has been set.

Lutein and zeaxanthin and eye disease: Scientific research shows that lutein can improve visual function in people with age-related macular degeneration. A high dietary intake of lutein and zeaxanthin has consistently shown to protect against age-related macular degeneration and cataracts. Currently, a large randomized controlled trial (AREDS-2) is studying the direct effects of lutein and zeaxanthin on the prevention of AMD.[19]

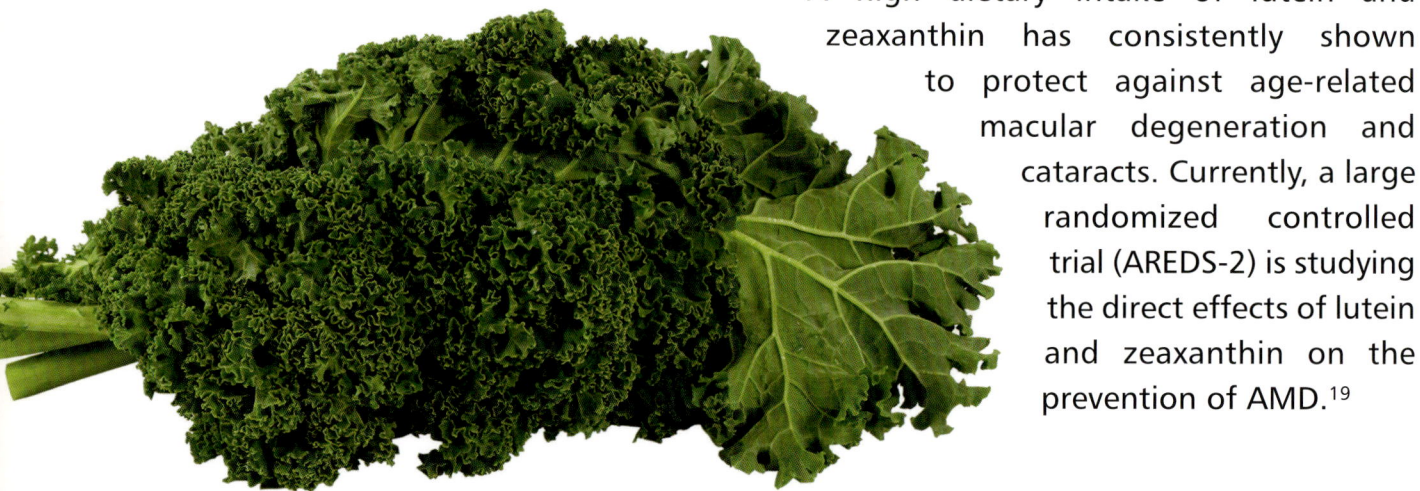

Part 1   The Basics

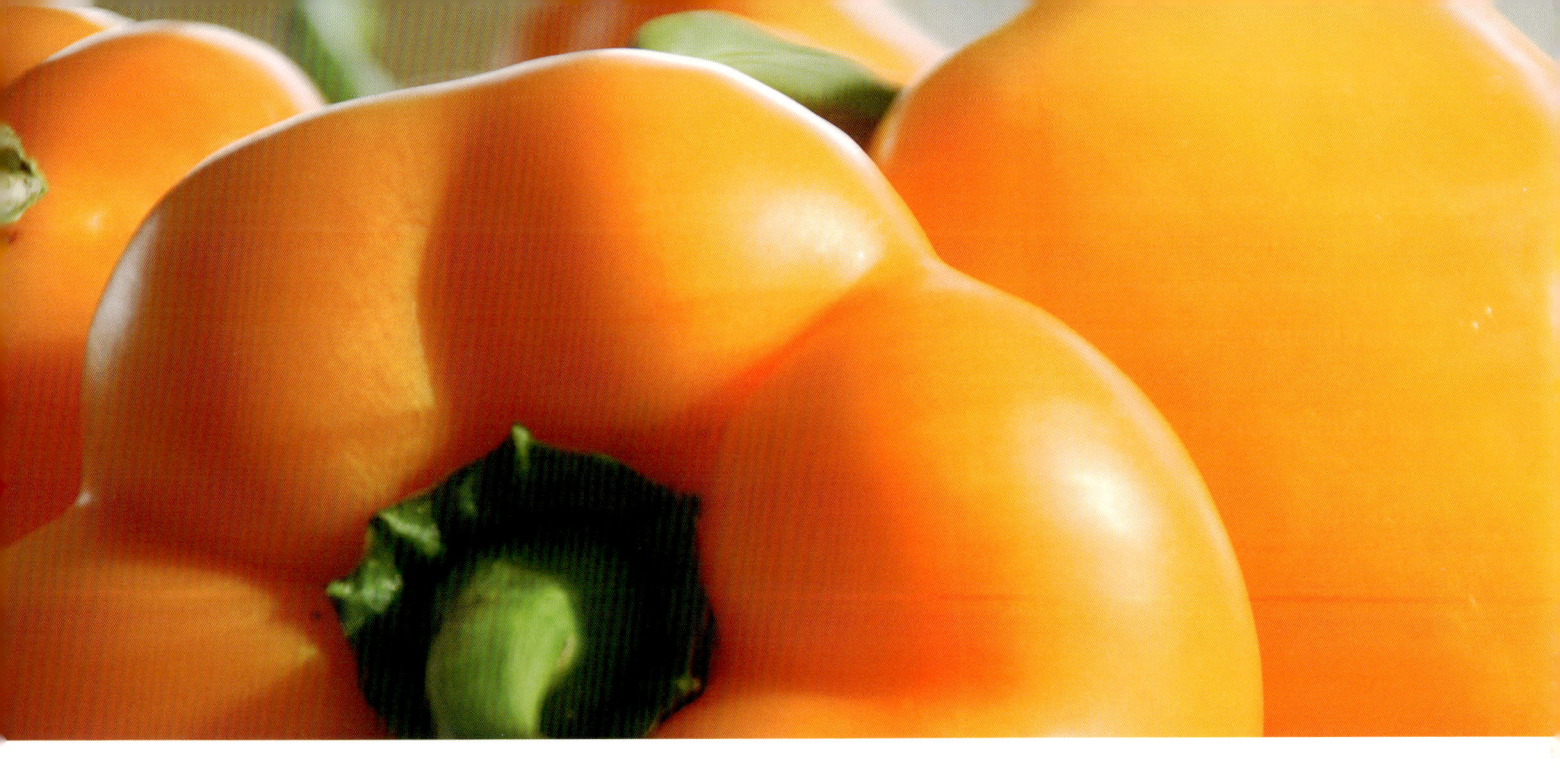

Lutein and zeaxanthin and general health:
Lutein and zeaxanthin are found in the skin and can help maintain healthy skin. They may also protect against cardiovascular disease and breast cancer.[20]

Vitamin C

Vitamin C (ascorbic acid) is a water-soluble antioxidant found in fruits and vegetables. It cannot be made or stored by the body, so it is essential to consume foods high in vitamin C daily.

Dietary Reference Intakes

RDA: Adult women – 75 mg/day
Adult men – 90 mg/day

UL: 2000 mg/day

Vitamin C and eye disease:
Diets high in vitamin C and other antioxidants have been shown to decrease the risk of age-related macular degeneration in elderly persons. Vitamin C can also decrease the risk of cataracts.[21]

Eye Nutrients   Chapter 2

Vitamin C and general health:
Vitamin C helps maintain a healthy immune system and increases the body's ability to absorb iron from plant foods. It may decrease the risk for stroke, heart attack, and lung cancer.[22]

Vitamin C supplements:
Effervescent vitamin C supplements are generally absorbed more quickly by the body than those in the chewable form. As the body cannot store more than 500 mg of vitamin C at a time, supplements of more than 500 mg should be taken twice daily.

Be aware:
- High doses of vitamin C (more than 2000 mg per day) may worsen symptoms in people prone to kidney stones.
- Taking more than 2000 mg per day of vitamin C can cause diarrhea, nausea, stomach cramping, excess urination, and skin rashes.[23]

Omega-3 Fatty Acids

Three important omega-3 fatty acids are DHA (docosahexaenoic acid), EPA (eicosapentaenoic acid) and ALA (alpha-linolenic acid). DHA and EPA are found in fish oils and ALA is found in nuts, flax seed, and vegetable oils.

DHA and EPA help decrease inflammation in the body. The body converts ALA into DHA and EPA, but as it is not an efficient process DHA and EPA are best consumed directly. However, ALA does have beneficial effects of its own, and should still be included in a healthy diet.[24]

Part 1   The Basics

Dietary Reference Intakes

AI (ALA): Adult women – 1.1 g/day
Adult men – 1.6 g/day

UL: To date no UL has been set.

Omega-3 fatty acids and eye disease:
Consumption of fish high in omega-3 fatty acids can decrease the risk of age-related macular degeneration. Both fish oils (DHA and EPA) and flax seed oil (ALA) are therapeutic for patients with dry eye syndrome.[25]

Omega-3 fatty acids and general health:
The American Heart Association recommends eating cold water fish at least twice per week, and that oils and foods high in ALA be included in a healthy diets. Fish oil has been proven to reduce the risk and severity of heart disease, high cholesterol, rheumatoid arthritis, and dementia.[26]

Omega-6 fatty acids:
Omega-6 fatty acids are unsaturated fatty acids that are abundant in the North American diet. They are found in vegetable oils, nuts, and seeds. People should strive to have equal amounts of omega-3 and omega-6 fatty acids in their diets.

Omega-6 to Omega-3 ratio:
Omega-6 fatty acids are pro-inflammatory and omega-3 fatty acids are anti-inflammatory. Our bodies require this opposition, but in the right proportion. Humans are thought to have evolved by eating a diet that provided equal amounts of omega-6 and omega-3 fatty acids (1:1). In our ancestors diets substantial quantities of omega-3 fatty acids were found in wild plants and wild game. Many natural sources of omega-3 fatty acids are now depleted, resulting in a change in our dietary ratios. In our current diets, omega-6 fatty acids are generally consumed over omega-3 fatty acids at a ratio of 15:1. Having a greater proportion of omega-6 fatty acids means that the body remains in an inflammatory state. We do need the pro-inflammatory component of the omega-6 fatty acids to heal from injuries, but once the healing phase is done, we

need the anti-inflammatory effects of the omega-3 fatty acids to return to a balanced state. Since the typical North American consumes many omega-6 fatty acids and far fewer omega-3 fatty acids, we need to focus on ways to balance the proportion by increasing our omega-3 fatty acid intake.[27]

Be aware:
- Certain fish and fish oils contain high levels of mercury. Health Canada recommends that pregnant women (and those trying to conceive), nursing mothers, and children should avoid eating fish high in mercury (shark, king mackerel, fresh tuna, swordfish, and tilefish). However, women should eat two meals per week of low-risk fish.
- Do not take more than three grams of omega-3 fatty acids per day unless under the care of a physician. High levels may cause excessive bleeding in rare cases.[28]

Summary of Omega-3 Fatty Acids (ALA, EPA, DHA)

Omega-3 Fatty Acid	Food Source
ALA (Alpha-linolenic acid)	Flax seed, flax seed oil, walnuts, walnut oil, canola oil, soy, wheat germ
DHA (Docosahexaenoic acid) **EPA** (Eicosapentaenoic acid)	Cold water fish, especially salmon, sardines, rainbow trout, mackerel

Part 1   The Basics

Vitamin E

Vitamin E is a fat-soluble antioxidant found in oils, nuts, eggs, some fruits and vegetables, and fortified cereals. Scientific studies show that vitamin E obtained from foods may be more beneficial than from supplements.[29]

Dietary Reference Intakes

RDA: Adult women – 15mg/day
Adult men – 15mg/day

UL: Adult women – 1000mg/day
Adult men – 1000mg/day

Vitamin E and eye disease:
Vitamin E, in addition to other antioxidants, may decrease the risk of cataracts and age-related macular degeneration.[30]

Vitamin E and general health:
Vitamin E has been shown to protect the body against cancer and cardiovascular disease. It works with Vitamin C to boost the immune system.[31]

Be aware:
- You should take vitamin E supplements under supervision from your doctor. One study suggests that 400 IU (international units) or more of vitamin E, taken daily, increases the risk of death in certain people. However, at lower doses, from diet or supplements, Vitamin E is not harmful.[32]
- As vitamin E is abundant in fats and oils, low-fat diets can be low in vitamin E.

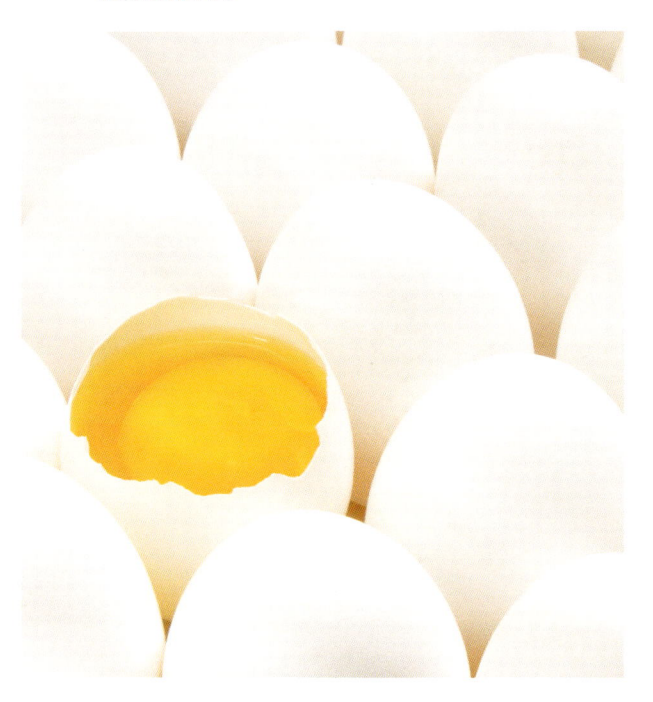

Eye Nutrients   Chapter 2

Zinc

Zinc is an essential trace mineral that exists in every cell of the body. It is found in seafood, meat, nuts, beans, whole grains, and fortified breakfast cereals. Oysters are the highest food source of zinc. However, North Americans get most of their zinc intake from red meat and poultry.[33]

Dietary Reference Intakes

RDA: Adult women – 8 mg/day
Adult men – 11 mg/day

UL: Adult women – 40 mg/day
Adult men – 40 mg/day

Zinc and eye disease:
Zinc intake from diet and supplements has been shown to protect against age-related macular degeneration. Antioxidant supplements with high doses of zinc (80 mg) are shown to decrease the risk of progression from intermediate to advanced AMD by 25%.[34]

Zinc and general health:
Zinc supports the immune system and the healing process, and it encourages normal growth and development during pregnancy, childhood, and adolescence. Zinc lozenges may decrease the duration of common cold symptoms.[35]

Be aware:
- Zinc toxicity occurs at 150 mg–450 mg/day. This can adversely affect the body's immune system, iron status, copper status, and HDL (good cholesterol) levels. There is no evidence of adverse effects from zinc that occurs naturally in foods.[36]

Beta-Carotene

Beta-carotene is a carotenoid found in fruits and vegetables. The body converts beta-carotene into vitamin A.[37]

Dietary Reference Intakes

RDA: To date no RDA has been set; however, the Institute of Medicine recommends consumption of carotenoid-rich fruits and vegetables.

UL: To date no UL has been set.

Beta-carotene and eye disease:
Beta-carotene may reduce the risk of progression of advanced age-related macular degeneration and cataracts when taken in combination with other antioxidants.[38]

Beta-carotene and general health:
Higher blood levels of beta-carotene may decrease the risk of chronic disease.

Be aware:
- People who smoke should not take beta-carotene in supplement form, as it may increase the risk of lung cancer.[39]
- Many AREDS-type supplements are available without beta-carotene for people who smoke.

Beta-carotene from food is generally safe. Over consumption can cause temporary yellowing of the skin, which is sometimes seen when excess carrot juice is consumed or when a baby is fed a large amount of carrot or sweet potato purée. This condition is harmless. When the body has enough vitamin A, conversion of beta-carotene to vitamin A stops.[40]

Eye Nutrients   Chapter 2

Vitamin D

Vitamin D is a fat-soluble vitamin stored by the body. As the natural levels of vitamin D in foods are quite low, many foods are fortified with vitamin D, such as milk and cereal flour. The body receives the majority of its vitamin D when UVB rays contact exposed skin, causing a chemical reaction that creates vitamin D. Less vitamin D is synthesized on cloudy days and during the winter. Wearing sunscreen with an SPF of eight or higher also limits vitamin D production.[41]

Dietary Reference Intakes

RDA: Adult men and women under the age of 70: 600iu/day
Adult men and women over the age of 70: 800 iu/day

UL: Adult men and women: 4000 iu/day

Vitamin D and eye disease:
Vitamin D may be associated with a decreased risk for early age-related macular degeneration.[42]

Vitamin D and general health:
Insufficient levels of vitamin D may increase the risk for osteoporosis by limiting calcium absorption in the body. Vitamin D may decrease the risk for certain cancers, heart disease, and type 2 diabetes.[43]

Be aware:
- Vitamin D supplements may interact with certain medications such as corticosteroids and cholesterol-lowering drugs.[44]
- From November to February in northern climates such as Canada, and the northern U.S., sun exposure alone cannot provide adequate vitamin D. The angle of the sun is such that UVB rays are limited, so even on a sunny day there will be little or no vitamin D production.

Fiber

Dietary fiber is the portion of plant foods that our bodies are unable to digest. It exists in two forms: soluble fiber and insoluble fiber. Diets high in fiber support a healthy digestive system.[45]

Part 1   The Basics

Sources of soluble fiber:
Oat bran, oatmeal, beans, barley, citrus, strawberries

Sources of insoluble fiber:
Whole wheat bread, cereal, cabbage, carrots, Brussels sprouts

Dietary Reference Intakes

AI: Adult women – 21-25 g/day
Adult male – 30-38 g/day

UL: To date no UL has been set.

Fiber and eye disease:
Diets high in fiber will benefit eye health in two ways.

- Diets with a high glycemic index can increase the risk of AMD and cataracts. Plant foods high in fiber tend to have a low glycemic index so are beneficial to eye health.
- The Heart and Stroke Foundation recommends a diet high in fiber. Supporting a healthy cardiovascular system also promotes healthy eyes.[46]

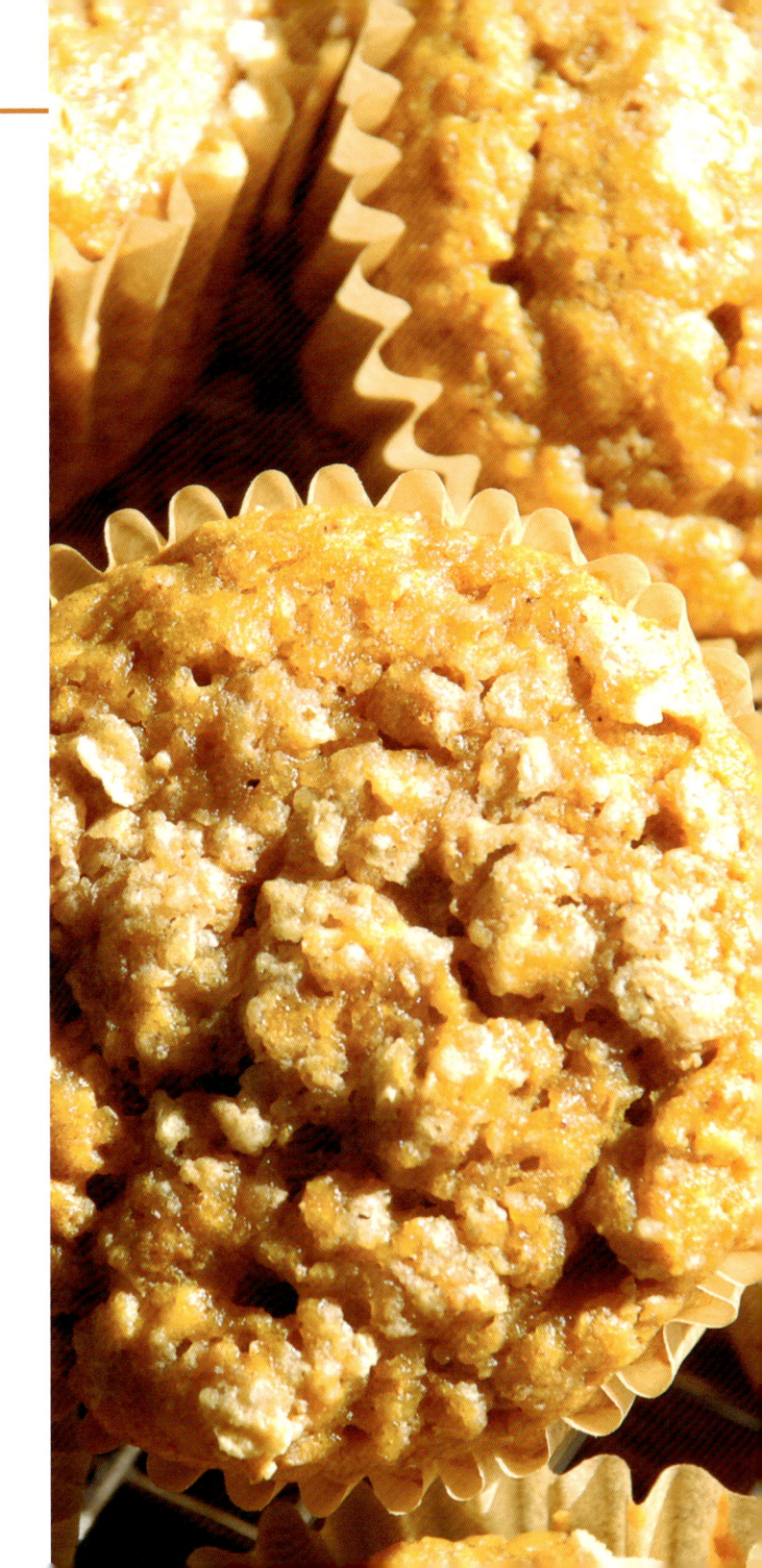

Fiber and general health:
When eaten as part of a heart-friendly diet, soluble fiber can decrease blood cholesterol. Insoluble fiber helps maintain healthy bowels.

Glycemic Index & Glycemic Load

Glycemic index:
The glycemic index is a measure of how much an individual food raises the glucose level in the blood as compared to a standard food (glucose or white bread). Researchers developed the concept of glycemic index for use in the management of diseases such as diabetes, where the body's glucose tolerance is disrupted. However, recent studies show the glycemic index of foods has a relationship to other diseases as well, such as cardiovascular disease, cancer, and age-related macular degeneration.

Foods with a high glycemic index include white bread, foods high in sugar (e.g. baked goods), and certain breakfast cereals. Foods with a low glycemic index include 100% whole wheat bread, whole grains (e.g. barley), legumes (e.g. lentils), and sweet potatoes.[47]

Glycemic load:
Glycemic load is a measure of the glycemic index of a particular food in relation to its carbohydrate content. This theory suggests that small portions of high glycemic index foods will have a similar effect on glucose levels in the bloodstream as larger portions of low glycemic index foods.[48]

Glycemic index and eye disease:
A diet rich in high glycemic index foods can increase the risk of cataracts and age-related macular degeneration. Low glycemic index diets will promote eye health.[49]

Glycemic index and general health:
Diets rich in high glycemic index foods can increase the risk of type 2 diabetes, cardiovascular disease, and certain types of cancer.[50]

Part 1   The Basics

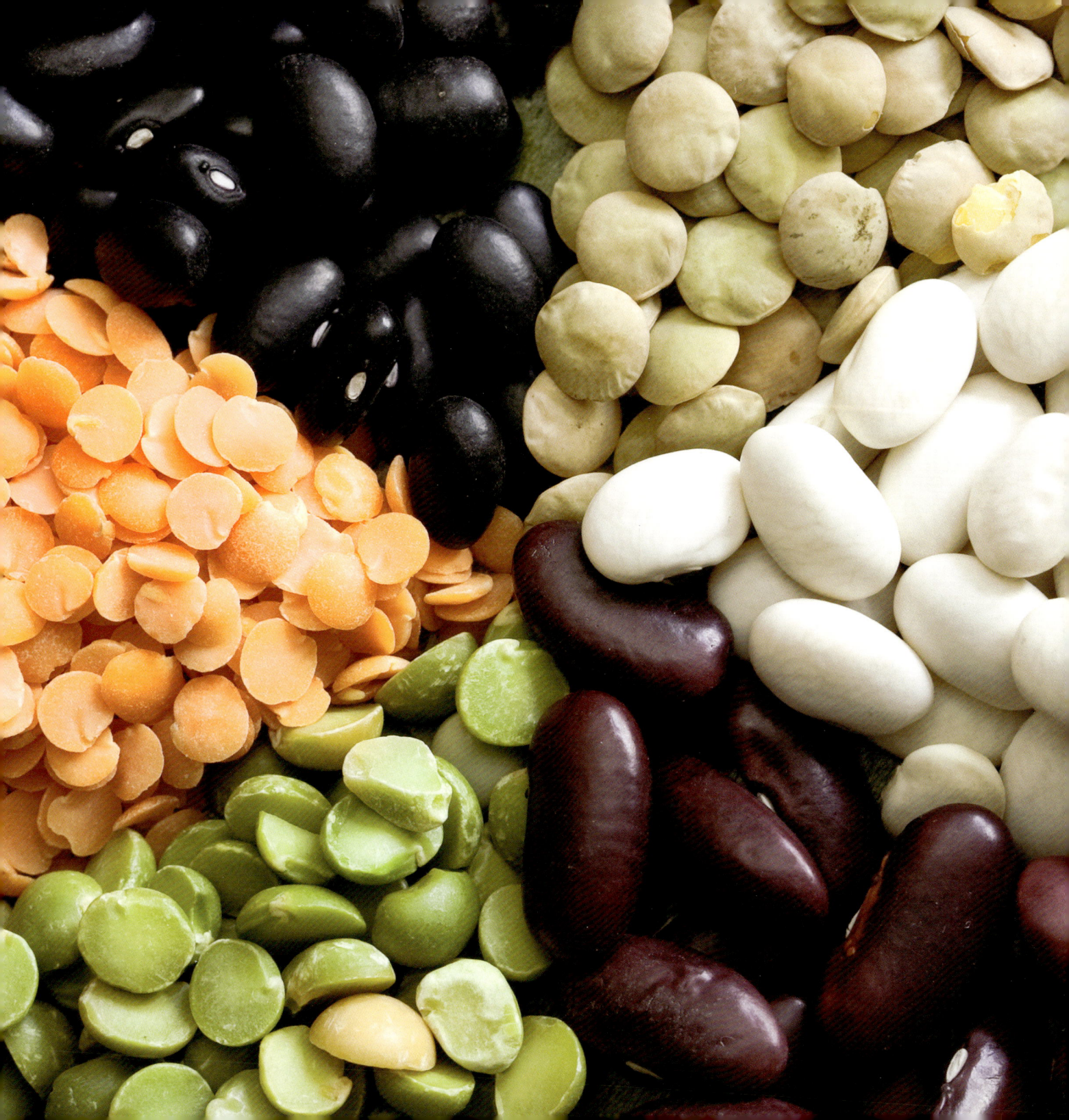

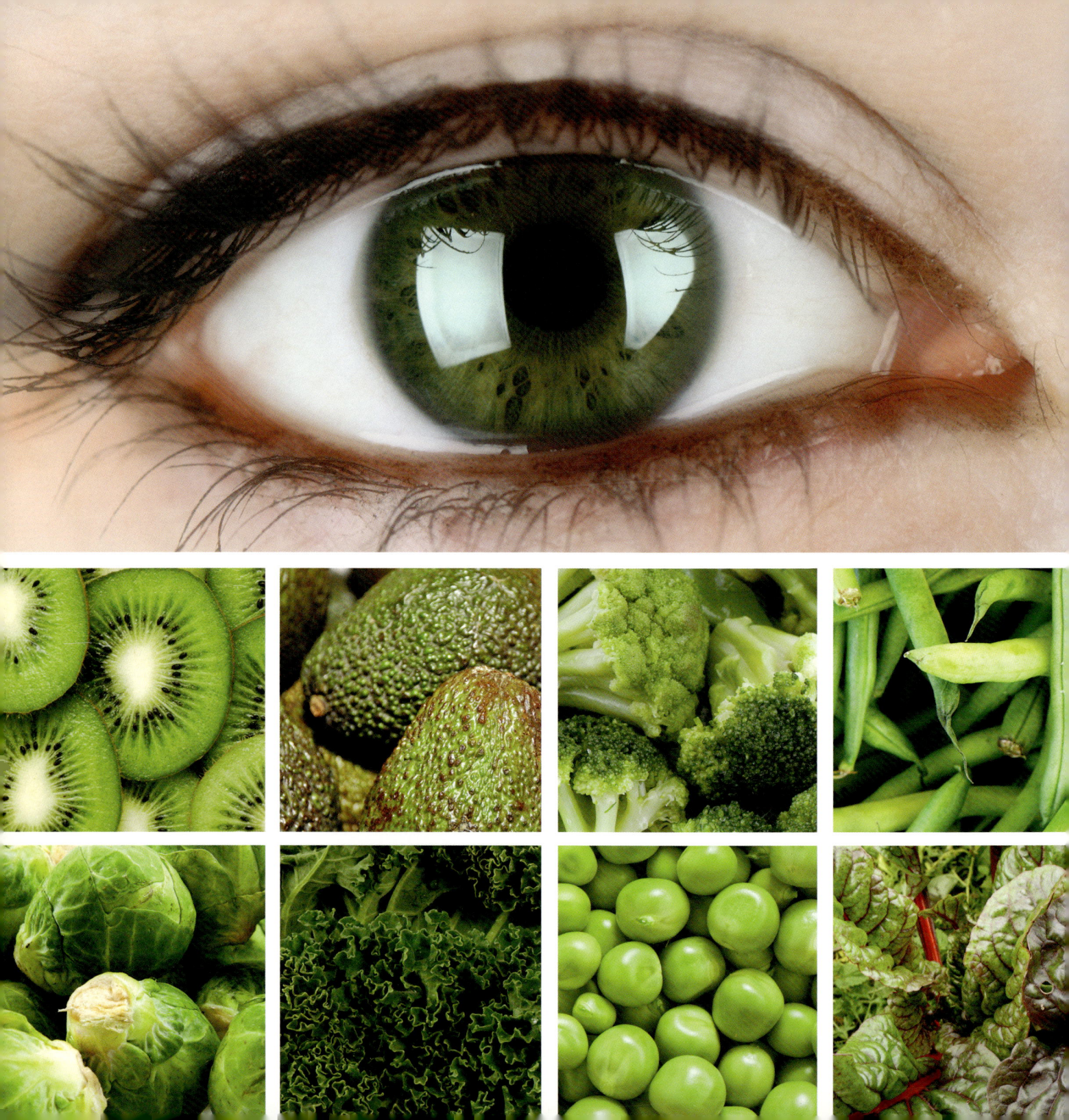

Part Two
The Details

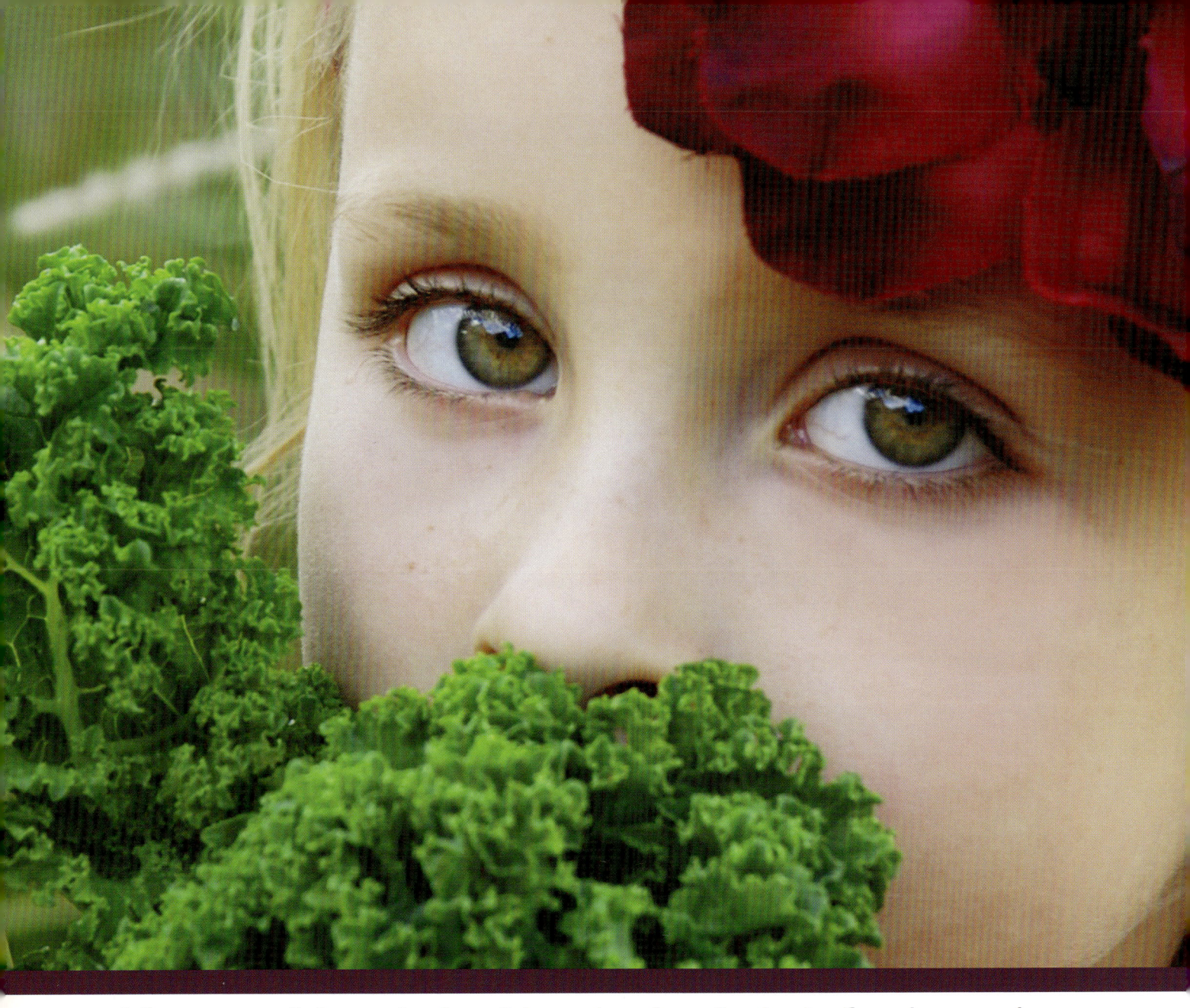

After careful analysis of hundreds of whole foods, we have identified the foods that contain the most eye nutrients. These are eyefoods.

Chapter 3
Eyefoods

A diet filled with the right foods helps to preserve eye health and fight eye disease. After careful research, we have selected the foods best suited to the promotion of healthy eyes. These are eyefoods, and they are loaded with nutrients that are beneficial to eye health.

After reviewing the nutrient content of hundreds of whole foods, we selected these eyefoods based on the amount and variety of eye nutrients they contain.[51] To obtain the greatest benefit from eyefoods, you should include as many of these foods in your diet as possible. You will be maintaining your vision and preventing eye disease, while at the same time decreasing your risk for cardiovascular disease and many types of cancer.

In this chapter, we will describe each eyefood and outline how each food promotes eye health and helps prevent eye disease. We will suggest a target for how much of each food to eat in a week, and we will give you valuable tips on how to integrate these foods into daily meals for yourself and your family.

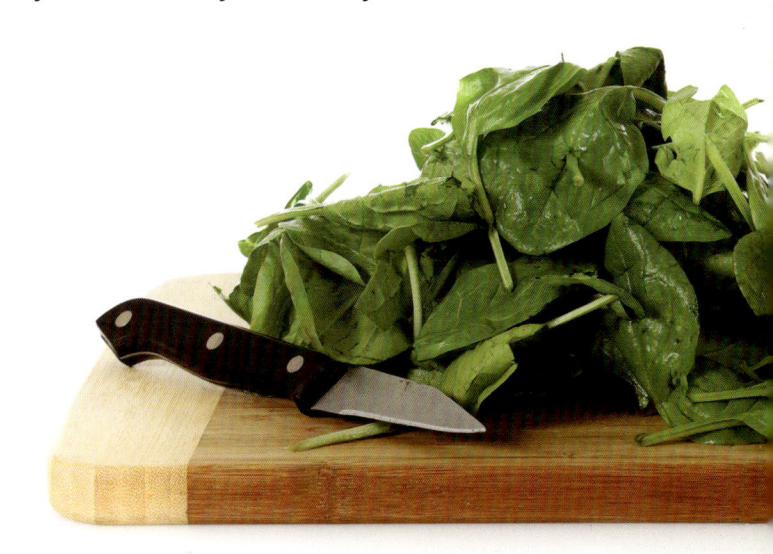

Leafy Green Vegetables

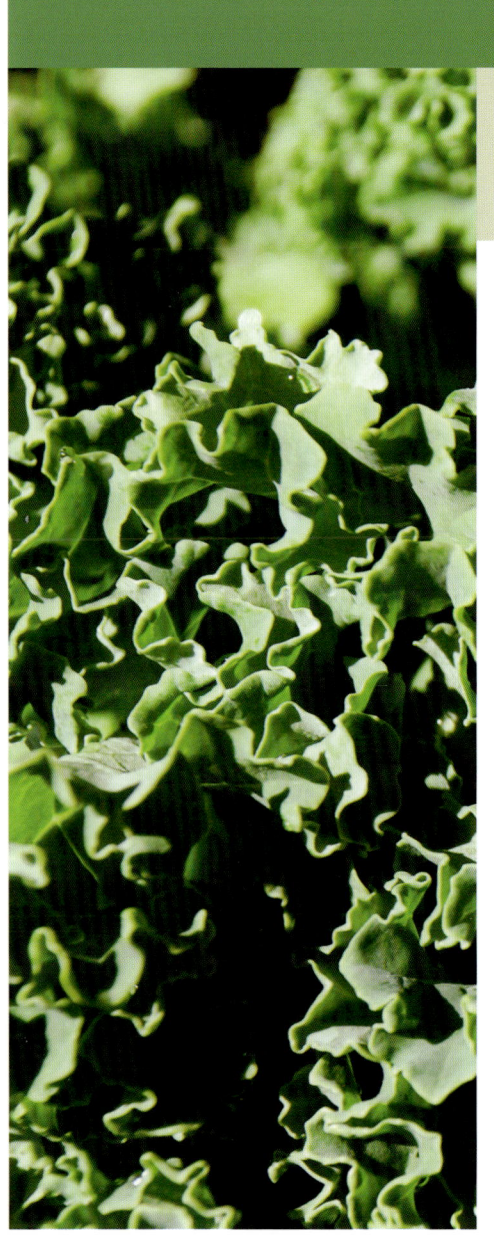

Kale, spinach, dandelion greens, romaine lettuce, radicchio, leaf lettuce, arugula, Swiss chard, rapini (broccoli rabe), collard greens

Eye nutrients:
Lutein and zeaxanthin, beta-carotene, vitamin E, vitamin C, zinc, fiber

Weekly target:
Raw: 1 cup or handful 7 times per week
Cooked: ½ cup twice per week

Overview:
Leafy green vegetables are the gold medalists of eyefoods as they contain most of the essential nutrients necessary for healthy eyes. Cooked and raw leafy green vegetables provide different nutritional benefits. When you eat cooked leafy green vegetables, the body absorbs more lutein and zeaxanthin, and when you eat raw leafy green vegetables the body absorbs more vitamin C. In addition to preserving eye health, diets rich in leafy green vegetables may decrease the risk of cardiovascular disease and many types of cancer.[52]

Part 2   The Details

Top Eyefoods: Kale, spinach, dandelion greens

Kale: This curly cruciferous leafy green vegetable is the number one food in this category. It contains three times the amount of lutein and zeaxanthin found in dandelion greens and spinach. If you eat merely one medium leaf of raw kale per day, you receive enough lutein and zeaxanthin to meet the eyefoods daily target. You can enjoy kale both raw and cooked, prepared in the same manner as spinach. Kale also makes a great substitute for cabbage in dishes such as cabbage rolls.

Spinach: Spinach and baby spinach are becoming more commonplace in the North American diet. We have known the health benefits of spinach for years. We all remember Popeye's bulging muscles as he consumed a can of this powerful green. Frozen spinach should be a staple in any freezer as this makes it easy to add it to dinners most nights.

Dandelion greens: Don't let its name scare you—this is indeed a gem of a leafy green vegetable. Eaten widely as a cooked side dish in Mediterranean cultures, one handful of dandelion greens added raw to a salad with leaf or romaine lettuce adds wonderful texture and a peppery flavor to every bite.

Eat a variety of leafy green vegetables: Each food in this category contains vital nutrients. Try sampling all of the different varieties to provide your body with the best nutritional benefits.

Enjoy them both raw and cooked: The nutrients in leafy green vegetables are available to the body in different ways depending on the state of the vegetable. For example, raw spinach is higher in vitamin C than cooked spinach, but cooked spinach is higher in lutein and zeaxanthin.

Eyefoods   Chapter 3

If your palate is not accustomed to the tastes and textures of leafy green vegetables, start slowly. Romaine and leaf lettuce should please any palate, while it may take time to enjoy the more intense flavor of kale, radicchio, or arugula. Add a couple leaves cut into bite size pieces to any salad. Don't be surprised if you come to love the intensity of their flavors.

Buy local: During the summer months, visit markets and farms to enjoy the flavor and freshness of local products. You can find spring-mix lettuce plants in most garden centers. Potted in your garden, this lettuce is a simple way for you to enjoy fresh, organic greens. During the winter, look for local radicchio.

Be aware: People on blood thinners need to watch their intake of leafy green vegetables. Blood thinners work by decreasing the activity of Vitamin K, which is abundant in leafy greens. Too many leafy green vegetables in a person's diet can decrease the efficacy of blood thinner medications and cause serious complications.[53] If you take blood thinners, discuss any potential changes in your diet with your physician.

Meal ideas

- Make a delicious tossed salad with mixed greens, citrus fruit, and walnuts.
- Sauté Swiss chard or any other leafy green vegetable with extra virgin olive oil, garlic, and salt and pepper for an excellent side dish.
- For extra flavor, sauté rapini (broccoli rabe) with extra virgin olive oil, add white beans, and season with salt, pepper, and hot chili peppers.
- Add frozen spinach to soups or omelettes.
- Grill whole radicchio leaves and drizzle with extra virgin olive oil.

💡 Tips

- Add extra virgin olive oil, canola oil, or walnut oil to cooked or raw leafy green vegetables to increase the body's absorption of lutein.[54]
- Try to incorporate at least two types of leafy green vegetables into your diet most days. For example, make a salad for two people with one handful of baby spinach and one handful of romaine hearts. The crispness of the romaine hearts will balance the smooth texture of the spinach.
- Have on hand one bunch of any leafy green vegetable per family of four every week.
- For quick and easy meal preparation, store washed, chopped, and blanched greens in the freezer.

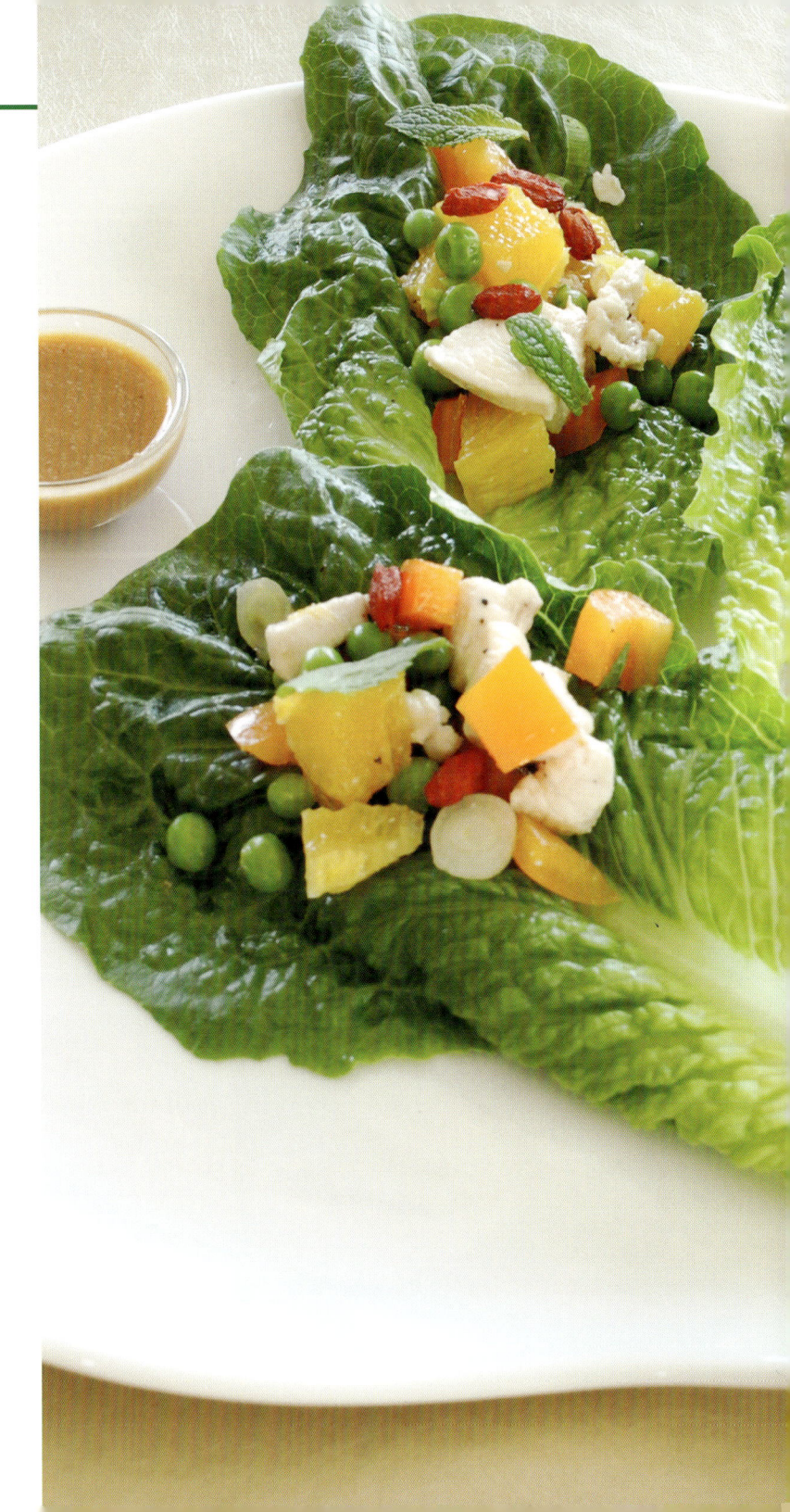

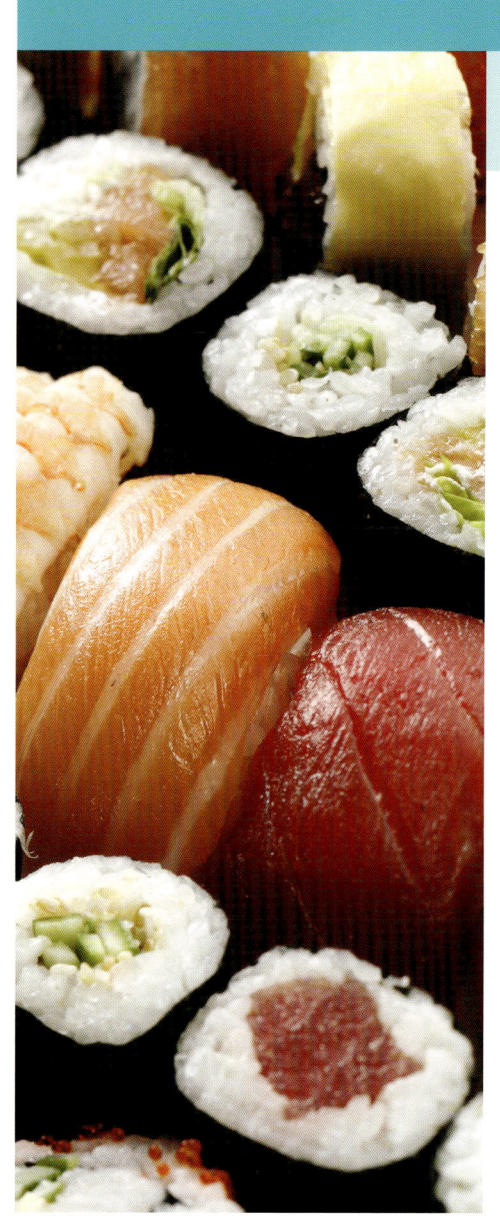

Cold Water Fish

Wild salmon, sardines, mackerel, tuna, rainbow trout

Eye nutrients:
Omega-3 fatty acids (DHA, EPA), vitamin E, vitamin D (in sardines)

Weekly target:
Wild salmon: 2 servings per week
Other cold water fish: 2 servings per week

Overview:
Scientists have found that eating cold water fish (fatty fish) has protective effects against age-related macular degeneration, cataracts, and dry eye syndrome. Omega-3 fatty acids found in fish may also decrease the risk of certain chronic diseases such as cardiovascular disease and cancer. The health benefits of fish make it an important addition to every diet. However, not all fish is created equal. Most fish is a great source of lean protein, but for the benefits of omega-3 fatty acids, some fish are a better choice than others. Wild salmon is a top eyefood because it has a high amount of omega-3 fatty acids. Other good sources of omega-3 fatty acids include sardines, mackerel, tuna, and rainbow trout.

Fish is abundant in Mediterranean and Asian cuisines, and it has important benefits for the cardiovascular system and the brain. Cultures in which people have a long life expectancy and lower rates of chronic disease often include fish as a dietary staple.[55]

Top Eyefoods: Wild salmon, sardines, tuna

Wild salmon: Wild salmon has a wonderfully rich texture and flavor. Its deep pink color and full-bodied taste distinguishes it from farmed salmon. Wild salmon is a better choice than farmed salmon because the mercury level of wild salmon is lower and the omega-3 fatty acid content is higher.

Fresh or frozen? Both are good choices. You can find seasonal fresh fish at most supermarket fish counters. It is always advisable to ask when the fish arrived to ensure its freshness. For optimal flavor and health benefits, the fresher the better. In the off-season, or for the sake of convenience, frozen wild salmon is also a great option, as the health benefits from fresh and frozen fish are the same.

Sardines: As a fish choice, they are one of the best. Some say that sardines are one of the healthiest foods around. Full of omega-3 fatty acids and vitamin E, they contain more vitamin D than almost any other food. As an added bonus, they are inexpensive and readily available in almost every supermarket. Sardines are popping up on the menus of the best restaurants, as their image is changing from a simple staple to more gourmet. In Mediterranean countries it is common to find fresh sardines, though in North America most sardines are canned. Sardines can sometimes be found in the freezer section of the supermarket. Try grilling them from frozen.

Eyefoods   Chapter 3

Tuna: Canned tuna is a staple in almost every pantry in North America. It is a convenient way to add fish to a busy lifestyle. Unfortunately, there are concerns over the mercury content in canned tuna. Health Canada recommends choosing canned light tuna over albacore (white) tuna because of its lower mercury content.[56]

How much canned light tuna should I eat? Health Canada does not offer any specific advice on the consumption of canned light tuna because of its relatively low mercury levels.

How much albacore (white) tuna should I eat? In 2007, Health Canada issued guidelines for the consumption of canned albacore tuna. Women who are pregnant, may become pregnant, or are nursing should eat no more than four servings (75 g or ½ cup) per week. Children between the ages of one and four should eat no more than one serving per week, and children between the ages of five and eleven should eat no more than two servings per week.

Be aware: Certain fish and fish oils contain high levels of mercury. Health Canada recommends that women who are or may become pregnant, as well as breastfeeding women, limit their intake of tuna (fresh or frozen), shark, swordfish, marlin, orange roughy, and escolar to no more than 150 g per month.[57]

The Blue Ocean Institute (www.blueocean.org) and The Monterey Bay Aquarium Seafood Watch (www.seafoodwatch.org) provide up-to-date recommendations on fish that is sustainable and safe to eat.

Canada's Food Guide recommends:
- Eat at least two servings (75 g each) of fish each week.
- Choose fish that are high in omega-3 fatty acids such as salmon, herring, sardines, char, Atlantic mackerel, and rainbow trout. These fish tend to be low in mercury.

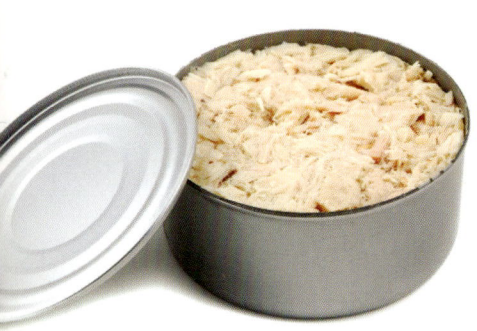

Part 2   The Details

🍽 Meal ideas

- Brush wild salmon fillets with olive oil, season with sea salt and black pepper, and bake at 375 °F (175 °C) for 15–20 minutes. Serve with sautéed or steamed leafy green vegetables.
- Make a high-protein salad with a can of boneless sardines, orange peppers, and sun-dried tomatoes.
- Make an attractive pepper boat with orange, yellow, or red peppers by cutting the raw pepper in half and filling it with tuna salad.
- Layer rainbow trout on top of a bed of thinly sliced lemons, onions and parsley in aluminum foil. Season with extra virgin olive oil, sea salt and pepper, and grill for 15–20 minutes on medium-high heat.

💡 Tips

- Buy one and a half wild salmon fillets per family member per week. Bake all at once for dinner and make a salmon salad with the leftovers to enjoy in a sandwich the next day.
- Give yourself a chance to develop a taste for sardines and mackerel by trying them every so often. Soon, you will find yourself reaching for them!
- Have a variety of boxed sardines and mackerel handy for an easy lunch. You can get skinless, boneless sardines and mackerel in different delicious sauces. Try a mustard variety for a quick and tasty sandwich.
- If you find it difficult to prepare fish at home, order grilled or baked fish when dining out at a restaurant.

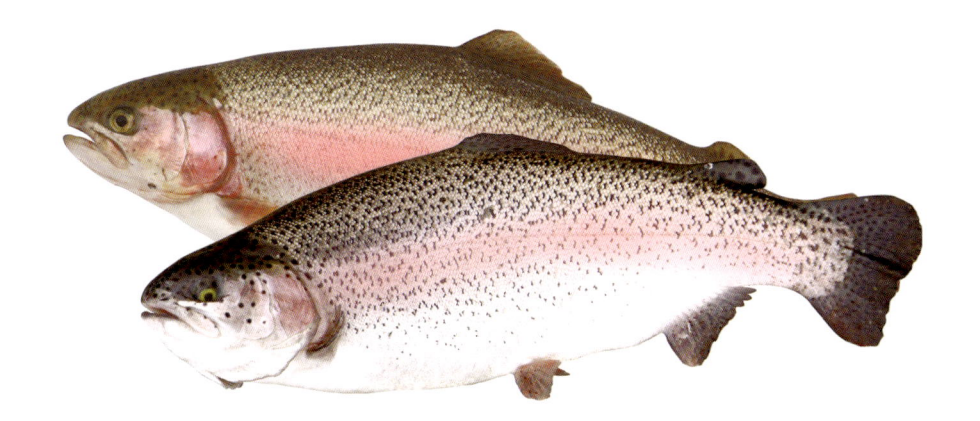

Eyefoods   Chapter 3

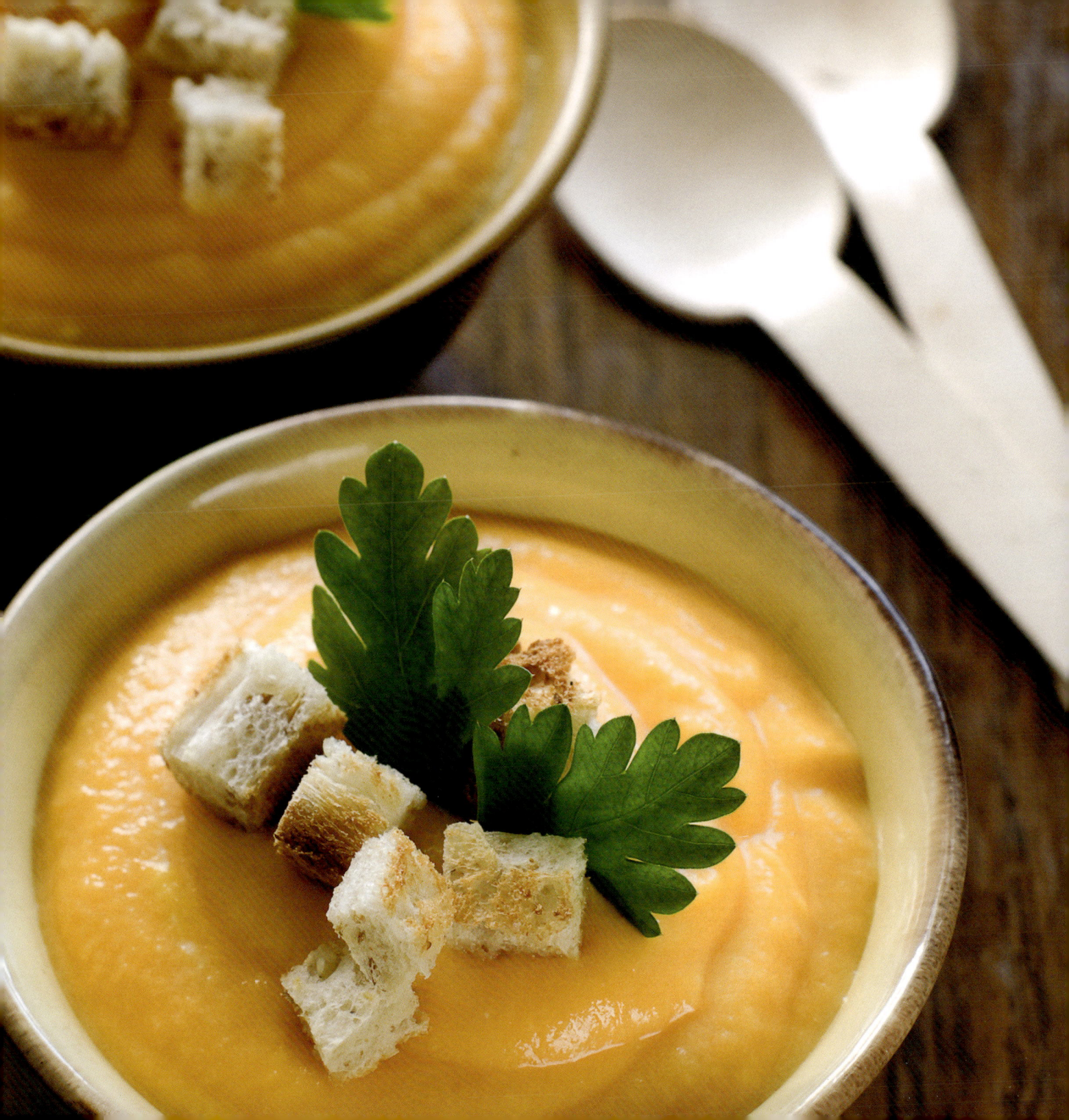

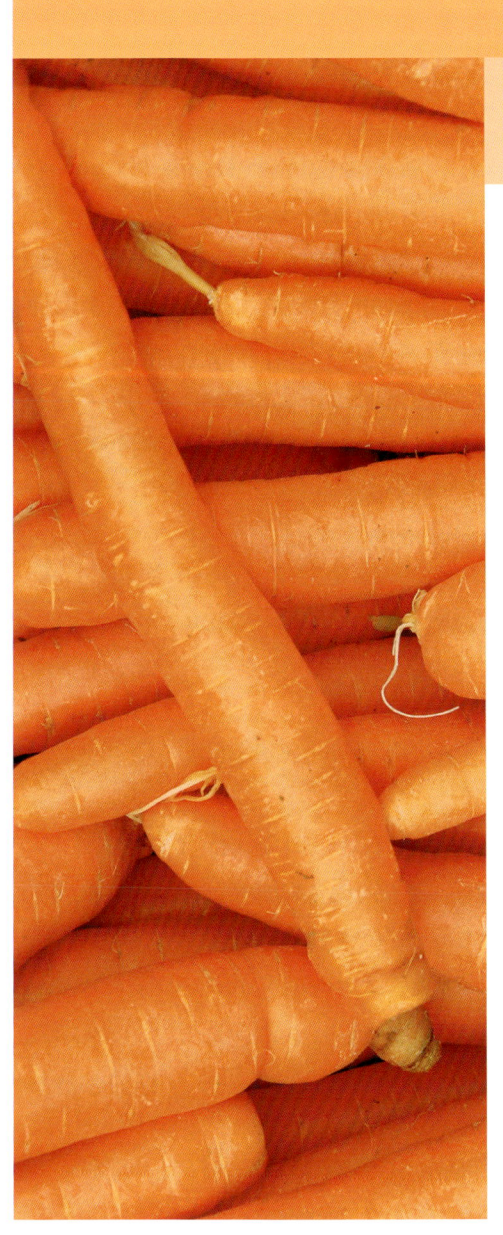

Orange Vegetables

Sweet potato, canned pumpkin, butternut squash, carrots

Eye nutrients:
Beta-carotene, vitamin E, zinc, fiber, lutein and zeaxanthin, vitamin C

Weekly target:
Cooked: ½ cup 3 times per week
Raw carrots: ½ cup 3 times per week

Overview:
Orange vegetables are the beta-carotene stars of the eyefoods. These brightly colored gems provide a bigger boost of beta-carotene than any other food group, along with significant amounts of most other eye nutrients. In addition to preventing eye disease, the antioxidants in these foods help to protect the body from diseases caused by oxidative damage, such as heart disease and cancer.[58] Research shows that beta-carotene supplements can increase the risk of lung cancer in people who smoke, so many AREDS-type eye vitamins do not contain this important nutrient. For this reason, an eye-friendly diet includes many beta-carotene rich foods.

Top Eyefood: Sweet potato

Sweet potato: Sweet potatoes top the list as the number one orange vegetable because they are the best food source of beta-carotene. They also contain a significant amount of fiber. They are readily available throughout the year in supermarkets and can be found in the late summer and early fall at local farmers' markets.

Eat a variety of orange vegetables: Eating a range of orange vegetables ensures you receive their maximum nutritional benefit. There are many different types of winter squash. Butternut, buttercup, acorn, and spaghetti squash are all great choices. Canned pumpkin is a convenient, healthy staple in any pantry. Be sure to buy 100% canned pumpkin and not pumpkin pie mix, which contains added sugar. Of course, we cannot forget to eat our carrots. Perhaps the most well-known and historic eyefood, carrots are inexpensive, versatile, and make a great snack. In addition, drinking carrot juice is a great way to get a beta-carotene blast.

Be aware: Carrot juice is best enjoyed in moderation. Consuming too much can cause your skin to appear orange.

Buy local: Sweet potatoes, carrots, butternut, and other winter squash are abundant in late summer and fall at local farmers' markets. These root vegetables store for weeks in a cool, dry place.

Canada's Food Guide recommends:
- Eat at least 1 orange vegetable each day
- Adults should eat 7-10 vegetable and fruit servings per day.

Tips

- Eat at least two different types of orange vegetables per week.
- Keep carrots in the refrigerator so that they are always available for a quick snack.
- Try eating the skin of the sweet potato, as it is loaded with vital nutrients and fiber.

Part 2   The Details

- Keep butternut squash in the freezer for a quick side dish to turkey or fish.
- Make canned pumpkin a staple in your pantry and add it to soups, stews, and muffins.
- Create delicious fall soups with any orange vegetable superstar. Top with crushed walnuts and enjoy.
- Make a beautiful centerpiece for your kitchen table or island with a variety of winter squash. Then they will be readily available to roast and enjoy.

Meal ideas

- Enjoy baby carrots as a snack with hummus or white bean dip.
- Sweet potatoes make a great substitution for white potatoes. Enjoy them baked, roasted, or mashed with a splash of extra virgin olive oil and a sprinkle of salt and pepper.
- Cut a butternut squash in half, roast, and drizzle with maple syrup.

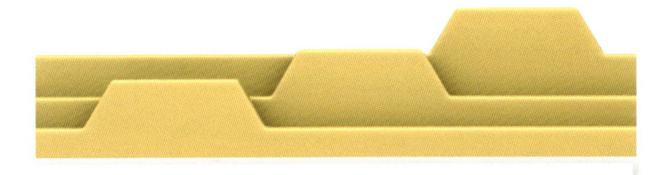

QUICK AND EASY RECIPE
Carrot Fries

4 carrots, peeled and sliced like French fries
2 tbsp olive or canola oil
1 tsp chili powder or paprika
Salt & pepper

Toss carrot sticks with oil and spices. Bake in the oven at 400 °F (200 °C) for 20–25 minutes or until cooked through but with a slight crunch.

Serve as a side dish or with a honey-mustard dip for a tasty snack.

Serves 2-3 people.

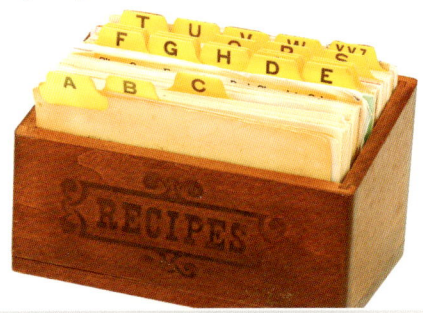

Eyefoods   Chapter 3

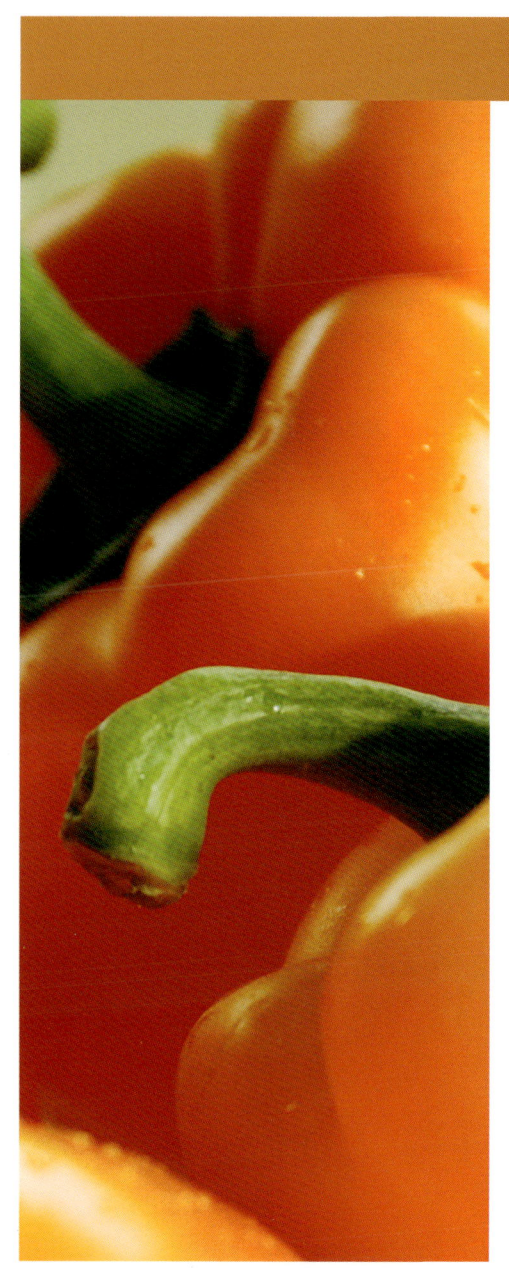

Orange Peppers

Eye nutrients:
Zeaxanthin and lutein, vitamin C, vitamin E, beta-carotene[59]

Weekly target:
½ pepper 4 times per week

Overview:
Of all the different colored peppers, orange peppers have the highest amount of eye nutrients. They are a high source of zeaxanthin, the macular pigment that acts as a sidekick to lutein. As we now know, lutein and zeaxanthin may reduce the risk of age-related macular degeneration and cataracts. In addition, just half of a large orange pepper contains nearly 50% of the eyefoods daily vitamin C target, making them the number one eyefood source of this essential nutrient. With higher levels of vitamin E than other vegetables, orange peppers are an excellent low-calorie source of the vitamin, which is more commonly obtained from fat and oils.

Don't let their color fool you. Although it may appear that they belong in the orange vegetable category, orange peppers stand alone as an eyefood. They actually contain only small amounts of beta-carotene. Their nutritional power comes instead from their high levels of zeaxanthin and lutein, vitamin C, and vitamin E. Eat orange peppers in addition to your other orange vegetables.

What about green, red, and yellow peppers?

Orange peppers have just the right mix of nutrients to make them an eyefood on their own, although yellow, red, and green peppers also contain high amounts of vitamin C. We recommend eating peppers of all colors, but when shopping for peppers, fill your cart with more orange peppers to get the most eye nutrients.

Meal ideas

- Enjoy raw orange pepper strips as a snack or as part of a vegetable plate
- Add chopped orange peppers to a spinach or bean salad.
- Cut an orange pepper in half or in quarters to make a pepper boat. Fill with egg, tuna, or turkey salad for a healthy lunch.
- Sauté orange, red, and yellow peppers with skinless, boneless turkey breast as a filling for a whole wheat pita or tortilla.

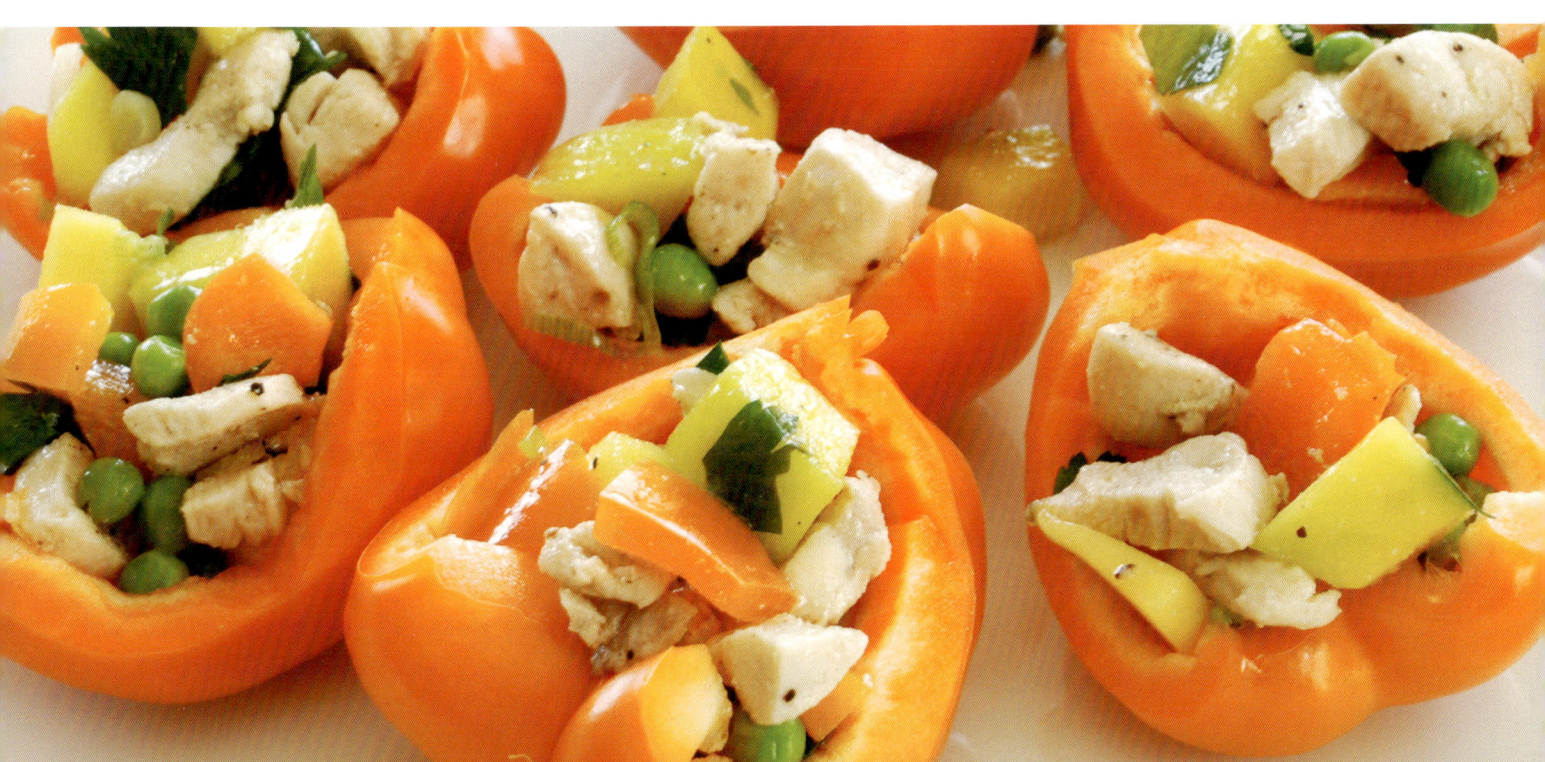

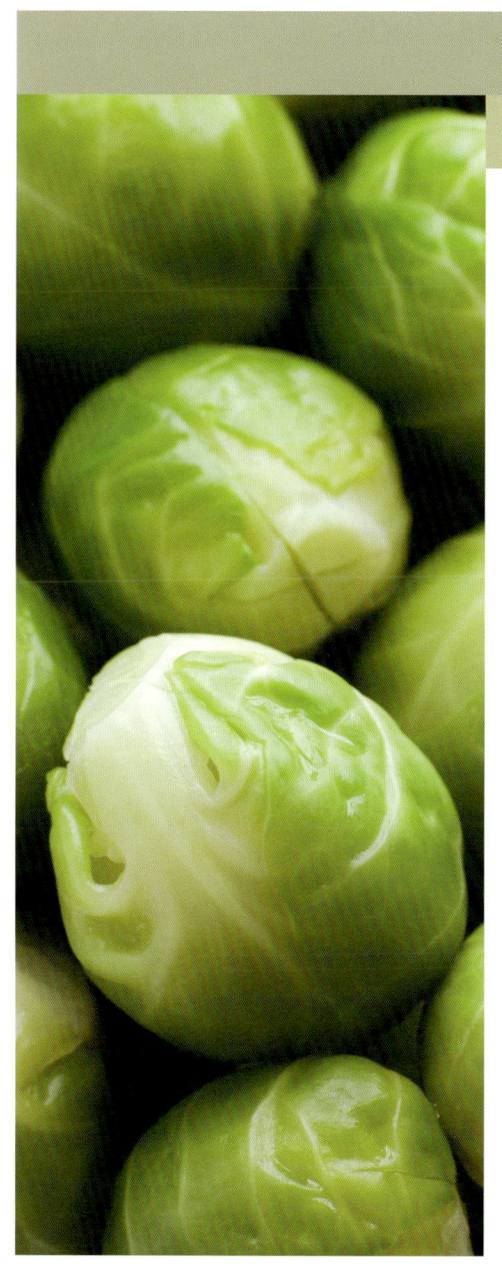

Green Vegetables

Brussels sprouts, broccoli, peas, green beans

Eye nutrients:
Lutein and zeaxanthin, vitamin C, vitamin E, beta-carotene, fiber

Weekly target:
Raw or cooked: ½ cup 7 times per week

Overview:
Each of the eyefoods green vegetables is high in lutein, zeaxanthin, vitamin C, and fiber. Raw broccoli is particularly rich in vitamin C, although cooking broccoli decreases the amount of vitamin C available to the body. Therefore, we recommend you include raw broccoli as part of your green vegetable choices every week.

You can find fresh Brussels sprouts, broccoli, and green beans throughout the year at the supermarket and locally grown in the late summer and early fall. During the winter, often select frozen vegetables over fresh. Fresh vegetables have to travel long distances to reach your supermarket, so the nutrient content will have decreased. Food processors freeze fruits and vegetables immediately after harvest when nutrient quantities are

Part 2   The Details

at their peak, so frozen vegetables maintain the majority of their nutrients. If you use canned vegetables, choose those without added salt whenever possible.

Canada's Food Guide recommends:
- Eat at least 1 green vegetable per day.
- Adults should eat 7-10 vegetable and fruit servings per day.

Tips

- Buy at least two different types of green vegetables each week, enough for two meals each.
- Gently steam enough green beans for two meals. Enjoy half the beans at one meal, and use the rest in a salad or to eat as a snack within the next few days.
- Have frozen peas handy for a nutritious last minute side dish.
- Thaw frozen peas for 20 minutes and add them to a green salad.
- Surprise your children with handfuls of half-thawed peas before dinner.

Meal ideas

- Enjoy raw broccoli with white bean dip or hummus.
- Make a colorful salad with raw broccoli, dried apricots, and walnuts.
- Steam Brussels sprouts or green beans with a little sea salt and a drizzle of walnut oil or extra virgin olive oil.
- Make a stir-fry with broccoli and lean beef. Add low sodium soy sauce, garlic, and pepper. Serve over barley or brown rice.

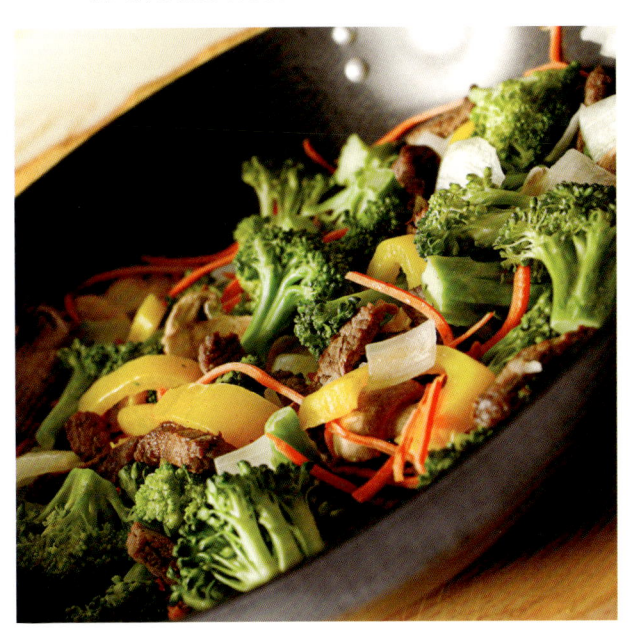

Eyefoods   Chapter 3

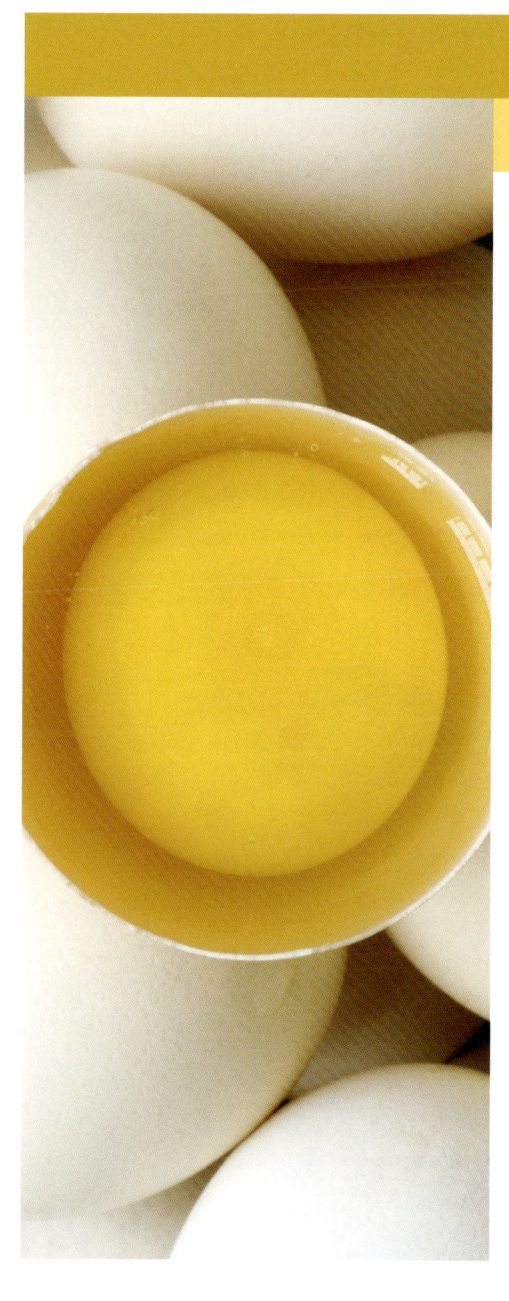

Eggs

Eggs high in omega-3 fatty acids

Eye nutrients:
Vitamin E, lutein and zeaxanthin, omega-3 fatty acids, zinc

Weekly target:
2 eggs twice per week

Overview:
An important eyefood, eggs contain significant amounts of vitamin E, lutein, and omega-3 fatty acids. Check the nutritional labels of the eggs and select those highest in omega-3 fatty acids whenever possible. Laid by chickens that have been fed a diet high in flax and corn, these eggs have a high lutein and omega-3 content. Eggs that are high in omega-3 fatty acids also tend to be a good source of vitamin E, and they contain a significant amount of lutein that is readily absorbed by our bodies.[60] Canada's Food Guide recognizes eggs as a healthy choice for lean protein.

Be aware: If you have a family history of heart disease or diabetes, or if you experience one of these conditions yourself, consult your physician regarding appropriate egg consumption.

Eggs: What's the story? Historically, popular media did not consider eggs a healthful food because of their cholesterol content. However, a large study published in the *Journal of the American Medical Association* in 1999 found that there was no link between moderate egg consumption (one egg per day) and an increased risk of stroke or cardiovascular disease in healthy patients. Further scientific studies have confirmed these findings. There does, however, seem to be a link between frequent egg consumption and an increased risk of heart disease in patients with diabetes.[61]

We believe that eggs, eaten in moderation, will provide the body with many healthful nutrients that ward off chronic disease and promote long-term eye health. Eggs are both healthy and delicious when boiled, poached, or scrambled, and they make a great meal as an omelette or frittata. Most of the egg's nutrients are in the yolk, so you should eat the entire egg for full nutritional benefit. Avoid cooking eggs in large amounts of butter or vegetable oil to limit saturated and total fat intake.

Tips

- Buy at least one dozen eggs per week for a family of four.
- If you enjoy egg salad as a quick lunch or snack, try using crispy romaine hearts or radicchio leaves in place of bread for an even more powerful lutein treat!

Meal ideas

- Enjoy boiled eggs drizzled with olive oil and seasoned with salt and pepper on a slice of whole grain toast for a nutritious breakfast or lunch.
- Make a delicious frittata or omelette with orange peppers and spinach.
- Serve bite-sized portions of frittata for a cocktail-party twist.
- Try making zabaglione, a classic Italian dessert prepared with egg yolks and topped with berries.

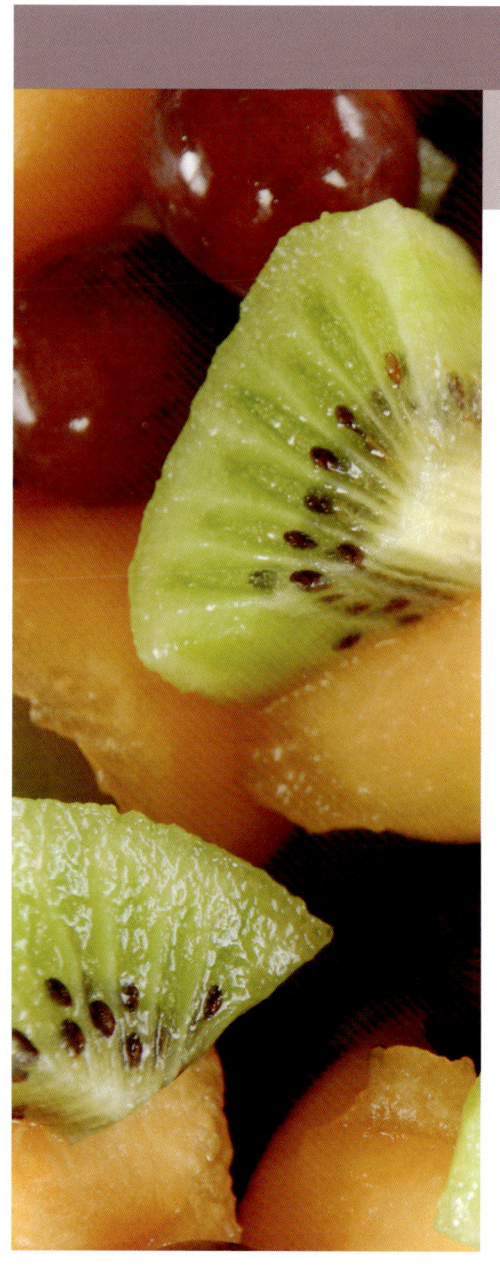

Fruit and Juice

Kiwi, cantaloupe, dried apricots, avocado (yes, it is a fruit!), berries, citrus, other fruits

Eye nutrients:
Lutein and zeaxanthin, vitamin C, vitamin E, beta-carotene, fiber, zinc, omega-3 fatty acids (avocado)

Weekly target:
Fruit: 3 servings per day
Juice: 1 cup of juice per day;
2 tbsp lemon juice per day

Overview:
Fruit and fruit juices are good sources of vitamin C. Since the body cannot store vitamin C, you should eat foods rich in vitamin C several times a day. Vitamin C is not the only nutrient you will get from eating fruit. Fruit is also full of other antioxidants that help to prevent disease. Enjoying a piece of fresh fruit can go a long way to satisfying a sweet tooth. We have identified kiwi, cantaloupe, and avocado as top eyefoods, although you should eat a variety of fruits to experience the greatest synergy of nutrients.

Part 2   The Details

Top Eyefoods: Kiwi, cantaloupe, avocado

Kiwi: The highest fruit source of vitamin C, kiwi is the top eyefood in the fruit category. Kiwi tastes best ripe, so when you are shopping for kiwi select fruits that are soft to the touch.

Cantaloupe: High in beta-carotene, cantaloupe is a versatile fruit that can be enjoyed with low-fat yogurt for breakfast or as a tasty dessert.

Avocado: Although not sweet, avocado has a beautiful creamy, nutty flavor and is a source of plant based omega-3 fatty acids (ALA), zinc, lutein, zeaxanthin, and vitamin E. Avocados are high in calories, so we recommend limiting avocado intake to half the fruit per serving.

Fruit juice: It is difficult to reach the eyefoods daily vitamin C target by eating fruit alone. Adding 100% fruit juice to your diet helps increase vitamin C intake. However, even unsweetened fruit juice can be high in sugar and calories, so enjoy it in moderation. Good juice choices include orange juice, apple juice with added vitamin C (ascorbic acid), and pineapple juice. Concord grape juice, pomegranate juice, and low-sodium vegetable cocktail are other good options.

Canada's Food Guide recommends:
- Adults should eat between 7-10 fruit and vegetable servings per day
- Have fruit and vegetables more often than juice

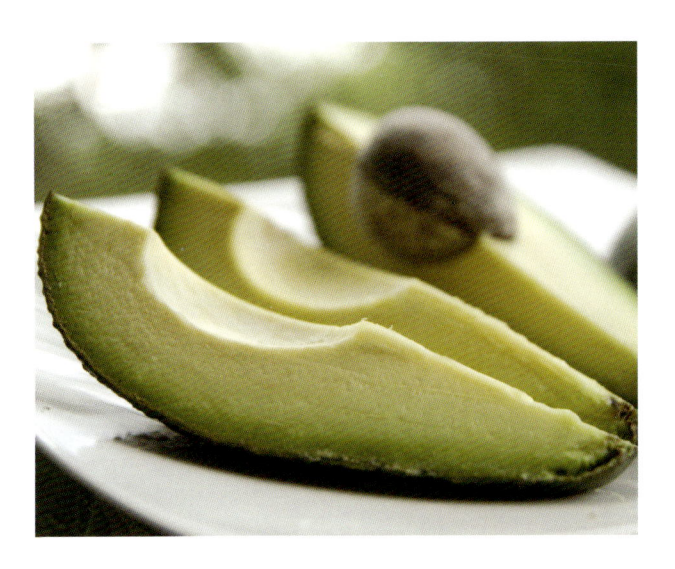

Eyefoods   Chapter 3

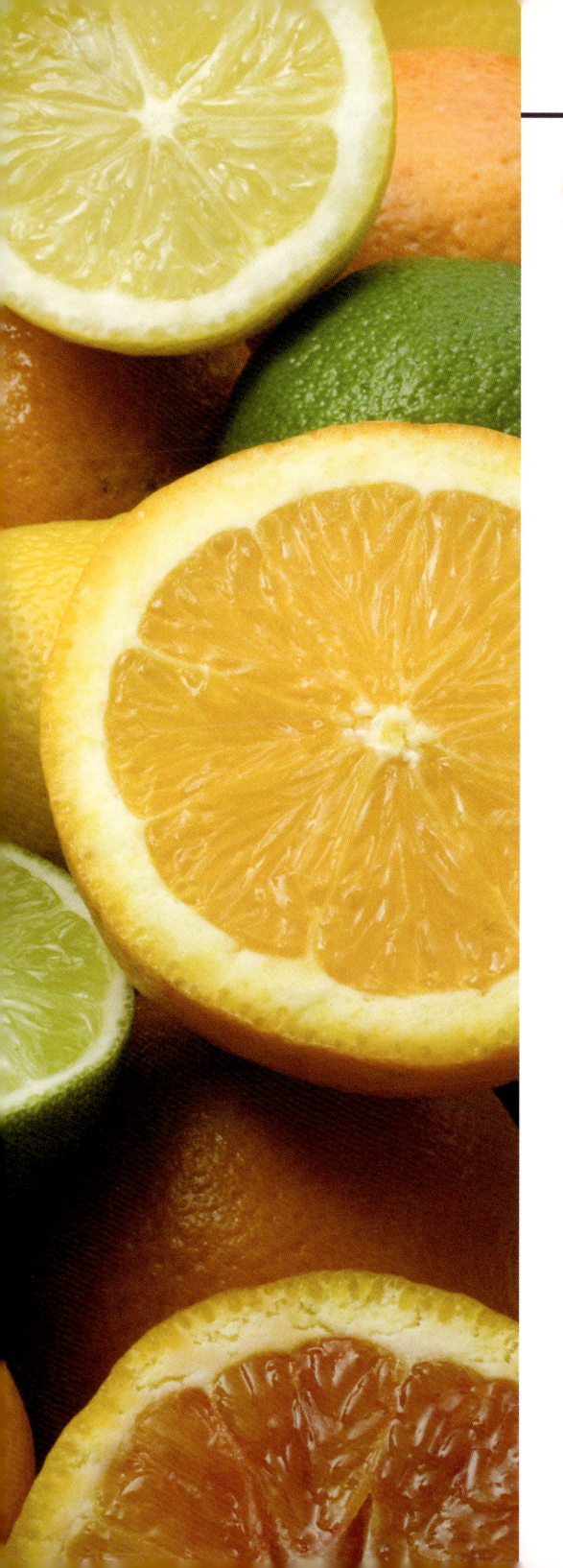

💡 Tips

- Start your day with fruit.
- Eat kiwis often—aim for one per day.
- A simple way to eat a kiwi is to cut it in half and scoop out the fruit with a teaspoon. You can also try eating the skin, as they do in New Zealand.
- Buy one cantaloupe every week for a family of four.
- Freeze sliced cantaloupe or kiwi when it is in season. Enjoy slightly thawed as a refreshing after-dinner treat.
- Add half an avocado to a grilled vegetable sandwich.
- Keep a jar of dried apricots on your counter and enjoy a few daily. (Dried fruit is high in sugar, so limit your consumption to four pieces per day.)
- Juice one lemon per person daily and dilute in water, tea, or juice, or pour over an avocado-and-crab salad.
- Choose freshly squeezed or frozen orange juice whenever possible.
- Choose canned or bottled apple juice over frozen apple juice.
- Create your own exciting juice combinations from left over fresh fruit. You can find affordable, good-quality juicers at most department stores.
- If you are trying to lose weight, limit your juice consumption.

🍽 Meal ideas

- Eat a kiwi each morning as you wait for your oatmeal or whole wheat toast to cook.
- Use a melon-baller to add cantaloupe for an attractive fruit plate.
- Treat yourself to an avocado-and-crab salad on a whole wheat pita for lunch.

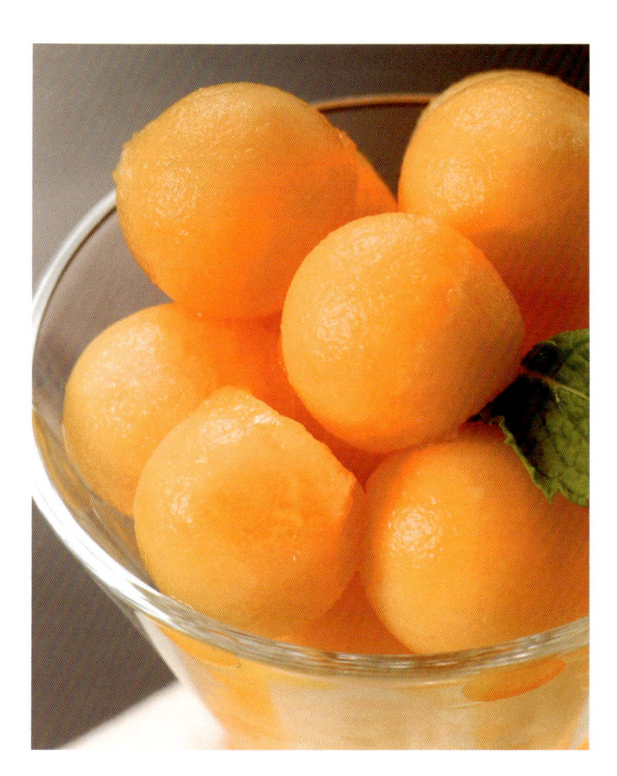

QUICK AND EASY RECIPE
Eyefoods Fruit Salad

½ cantaloupe
1 cup red grapes
2 kiwis, peeled
1 lime, juiced
1 tbsp maple syrup
¼ cup goji berries or dried cranberries

Cut a cantaloupe in half. Using a melon baller, make balls out of the cantaloupe. Cut the kiwi in four lengthwise, then cut each quarter in four, creating quarter circles. Place all fruit in a serving bowl. Mix lime juice and maple syrup and stir gently into the fruit bowl. Serve and garnish with goji berries or dried cranberries.

Serves 4.

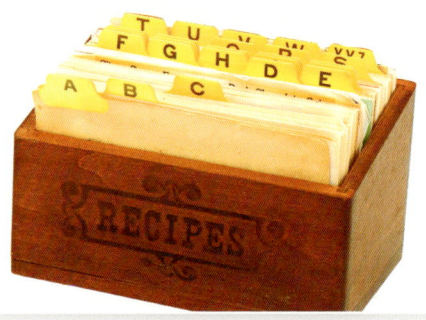

Eyefoods   Chapter 3

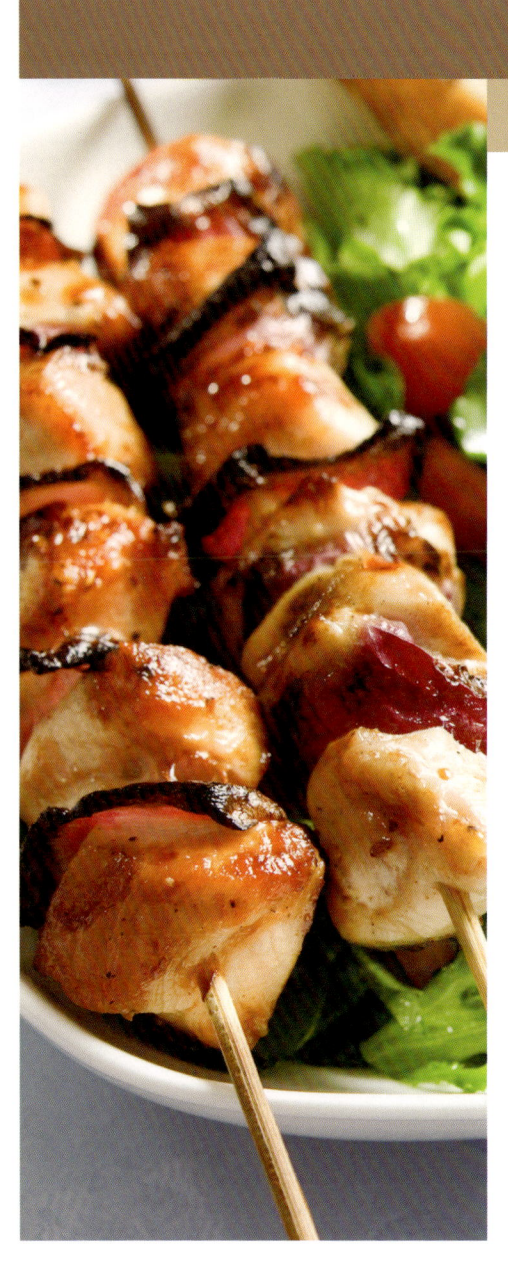

Lean Protein

Turkey, lean cuts of beef, seafood

Eye nutrients:
Zinc, vitamin E, omega-3 fatty acids (DHA, EPA)

Weekly target:
Turkey breast: 100 g – 4 times per week
Lean cuts of beef: 100 g – 2 times per week

Overview:
Turkey breast and lean beef are important eyefoods because they contain large amounts of zinc and vitamin E. It is easier to achieve an optimal daily intake of zinc and vitamin E from your diet if you consume some lean meat, fish, or seafood. Certain meats can be high in saturated fat, so we recommend choosing leaner cuts, limiting portion sizes, and removing the skin from turkey and chicken. It is recommended that you limit the consumption of meat, poultry, and fish to no more than six cooked ounces (170g) per day.[62] A three-ounce portion is approximately the size of a deck of playing cards.

Other meats and seafood that are good choices for lean protein are canned crab, dark turkey meat, chicken, oysters, clams, and scallops.

Part 2   The Details

Be aware: It is difficult for a person to achieve the recommended daily allowance of zinc without consuming some meat or seafood, so vegetarians need to carefully monitor their zinc intake.

Canada's Food Guide recommends:
- Adults should eat 2-3 servings (75 g per serving) of meat and alternatives per day.
- Trim the visible fat from meats and remove the skin on poultry. Roast, bake, or poach food and use little or no added fat.

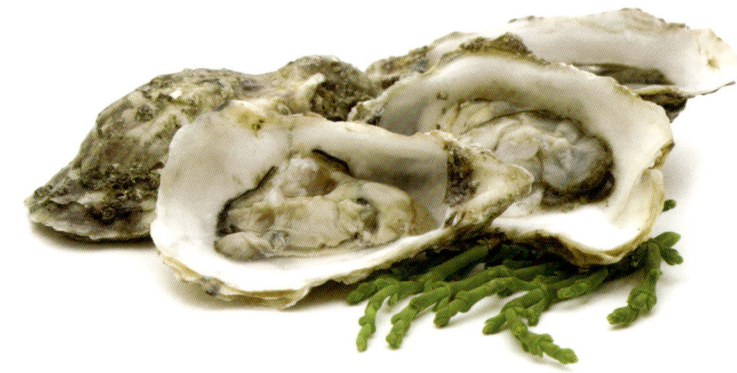

- Use canned crab as you would use canned tuna or salmon. Add it to salads and pastas or use it to make a quick, flavorful dip.
- Eat cooked or smoked oysters occasionally. They top the eyefoods for zinc!

💡 Tips

- Use turkey breast fillets in place of chicken breasts. The zinc content is much greater in turkey than in chicken.
- Don't reserve turkey dinners for holidays. Roast a turkey for a great Sunday meal with lots of left overs.
- Use ground turkey instead of ground beef for healthier hamburgers, meatballs, or chili.

🍽 Meal ideas

- Make a sandwich with turkey breast, whole grain bread, sliced apples, Swiss cheese, arugula, and Dijon mustard. Grill in a panini press or on the stove. Drizzle with balsamic glaze.
- Sprinkle canned crab over low-fat cream cheese and seafood sauce for a tasty dip. Enjoy with baby carrots or whole grain pita toasts.

Eyefoods   Chapter 3

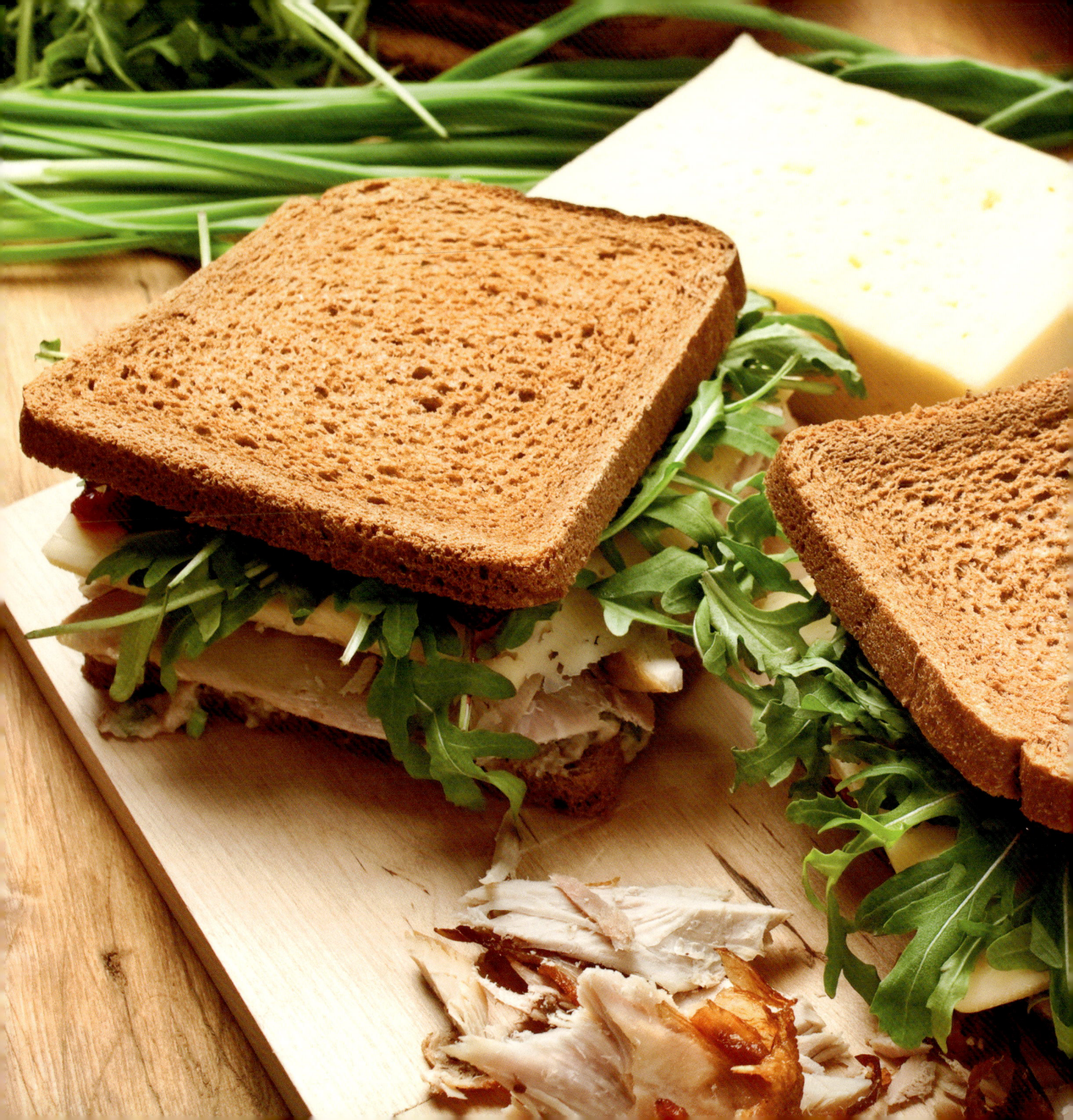

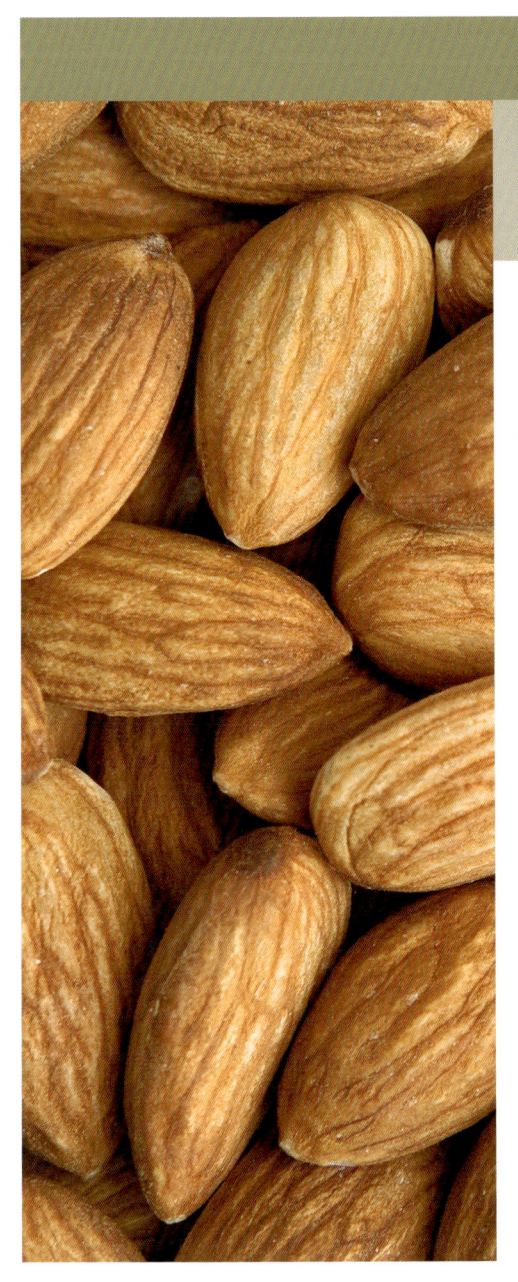

Nuts and Seeds

Almonds, walnuts, cashews, sunflower seeds, pumpkin seeds, pistachios, hazelnuts, pine nuts, pecans, dry-roasted soybeans

Eye nutrients:
Fiber, omega-3 fatty acids, vitamin E, zinc

Weekly target:
Eyefoods nut mix: 1 small handful per day
Ground flax seed or wheat germ: 1 tablespoon per day

Overview:
These nutrient-rich nibbles are powerful eyefoods that contain generous amounts of eye nutrients. In fact, eating nuts may protect against the progression of age-related macular degeneration, cardiovascular disease, and type 2 diabetes.[63] As each nut and seed has its own nutritional benefit, we recommend eating a good variety. To enjoy a healthy selection of nuts, simply prepare the eyefoods nut mix recipe described on page 97 and eat one small handful (about 1/4 cup) per day. This nut mix contains a balanced amount of vitamin E, zinc, and omega-3 fatty acids (ALA).

Eyefoods   Chapter 3

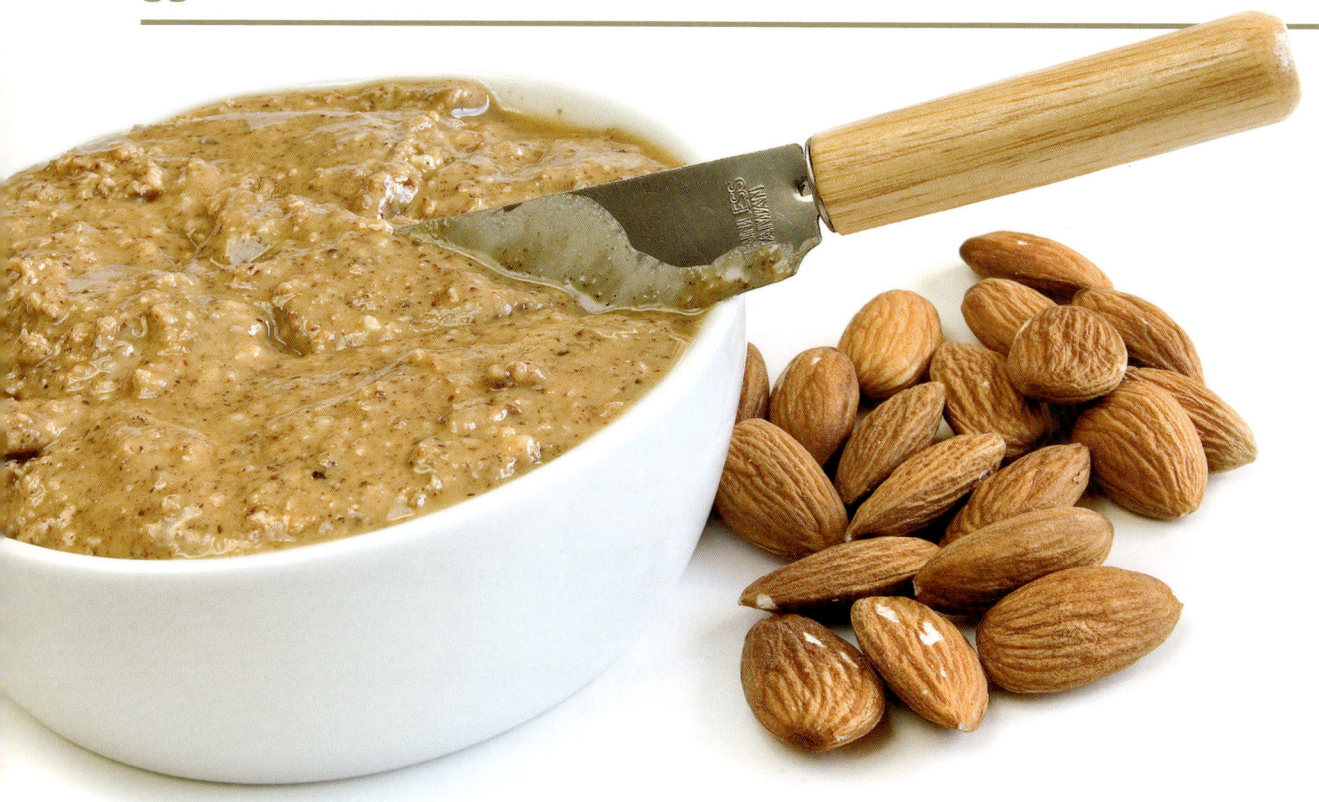

What kinds of nuts and seeds should I buy? Unsalted, raw, or dry-roasted nuts are best. If you buy large quantities of nuts at a time, freeze them to prevent oxidation, which gives them a rancid taste and decreases their nutrient content. Many different varieties of nuts are available in the bulk section of most supermarkets. Raw cashews and peanuts can be found in health food or bulk food stores.

Nut butters: Nutritious and tasty, nut butters are a convenient way for you to enjoy the health benefits of nuts. We recommend unsweetened and natural peanut, almond, and cashew butters. All are available in most supermarkets and health food stores.

Part 2   The Details

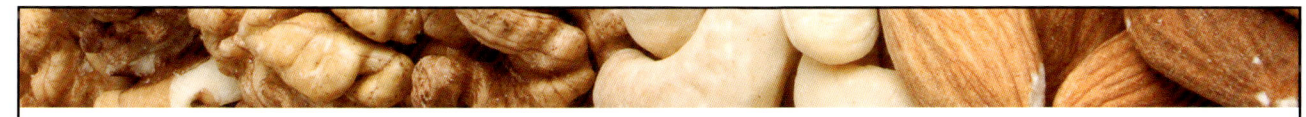

Top Eyefoods: Almonds, walnuts, cashews, sunflower seeds, pumpkin seeds

Nut or Seed	Key Eye Nutrient
Almonds	Vitamin E
Walnuts	Omega-3 fatty acid (ALA)
Cashews	Zinc
Sunflower seeds	Vitamin E
Pumpkin seeds	Zinc

Be aware:
- Nuts and nut butters are high in calories, so consume only one handful of nuts or two tablespoons of nut butter per day.
- We advise that you reduce your fat intake from other sources when adding nuts to your diet. What is the best way to eliminate excess fats? Reduce your meat, butter, or margarine intake.

Canada's Food Guide recommends:
- Nuts are included in the "Meat and Alternatives" category. Adults should eat 2-3 servings of meat and alternatives per day.
- One handful (1/4 cup) of nuts is equal to one serving.

Eyefoods   Chapter 3

💡 Tips

- Make a trail mix with a variety of nuts, seeds, and dried apricots.
- Make a decadent hazelnut spread by mixing hazelnut butter with a little cocoa, milk, and honey.
- Before adding to a salad or rice bowl, toast nuts in a dry frying pan for a few minutes to enhance their flavor.
- Buy fresh nuts in their shells in late fall and winter. Enjoy them with the family after dinner as a fun treat.

🍽 Meal ideas

- Eat nuts with your breakfast to include protein in the first meal of the day. The protein kick will delay mid-morning hunger that can lead to snacking on less nutritious foods.
- Add walnuts and almonds to brown rice for a creative side dish.
- Make a home made pesto sauce by mixing pine nuts with extra virgin olive oil, garlic, and basil in a food processor or blender. Mix the pesto sauce with whole wheat pasta or use it as a spread on whole wheat bread.

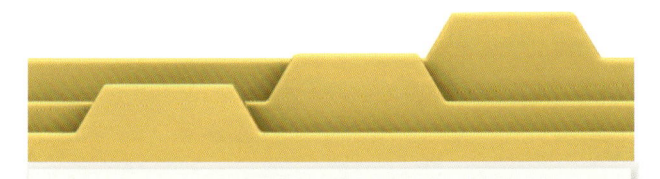

QUICK AND EASY RECIPE

Eyefoods Nut Mix

1 cup chopped almonds
½ cup chopped walnuts
1 cup chopped cashews
1 cup pumpkin seeds

Mix all ingredients in a large bowl. Transfer to a glass jar or storage container. Store in the refrigerator for 2-4 weeks.

Makes 3 ½ cups.

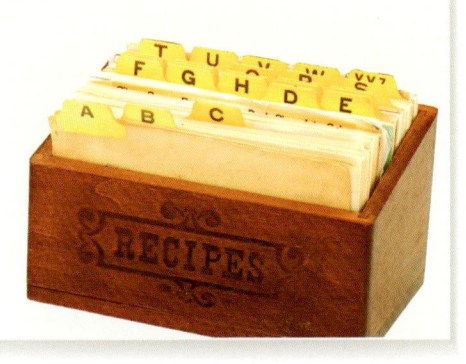

Part 2   The Details

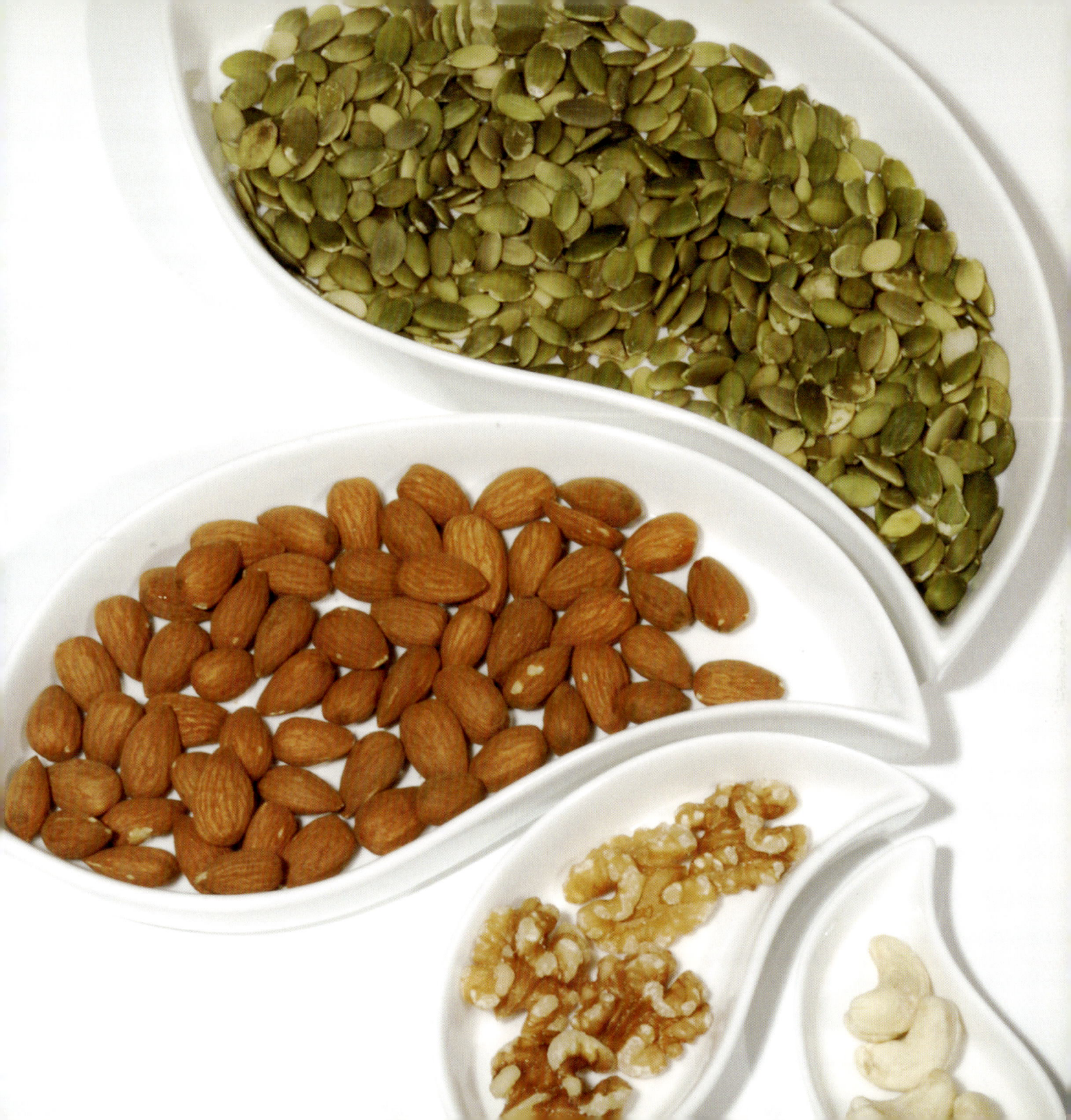

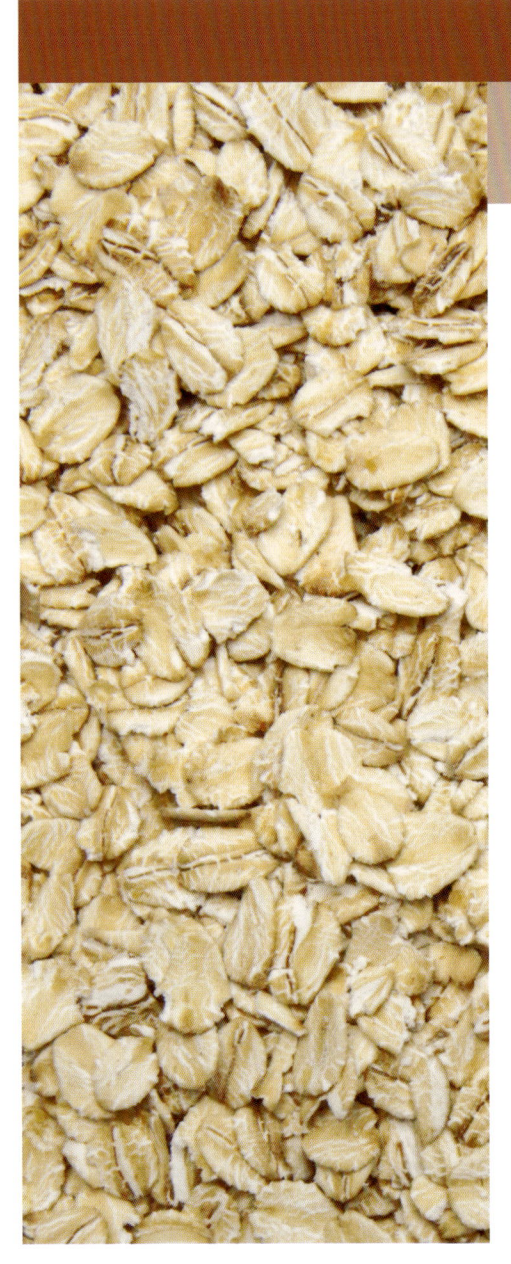

Whole Grains

Bran cereal, oatmeal, barley, whole wheat pasta, quinoa, other whole grains

Eye nutrients:
Fiber, zinc, vitamin E

Weekly target:
1 small bowl (3/4 cup) of bran cereal or oatmeal 5 times per week. Eat a variety of other whole grains following Canada's Food Guide.

Overview:
Whole grains are an important eyefood because of their high fiber content and a low glycemic index. Current research shows that diets rich in foods with a high glycemic index such as white bread and sugar can increase the risk of cataracts and age-related macular degeneration. As much as possible, choose whole grain foods over refined carbohydrates such as white bread, white rice or pasta.[64]

The British Journal of Ophthalmology published a study in 2008 showing that people with age-related macular degeneration have a higher risk of developing cardiovascular disease.[65] Because age-related macular degeneration and cardiovascular disease share many

Part 2   The Details

common risk factors, we believe that a heart-friendly diet is an eye-friendly diet, and that increasing your fiber intake will contribute to healthy blood vessels and eyes.

Top Eyefoods: Bran cereal, oatmeal

To achieve the recommended daily allowance for fiber (approximately 25 grams per day for women and 35 grams per day for men), we recommend eating bran cereal and oatmeal on a regular basis. Beginning your day with bran cereal or oatmeal will also curb mid-morning hunger.

Bran cereal: Bran cereal is high in fiber and has a low glycemic index. Try to choose bran cereal that has a high fiber content and minimal added sugar.

Oatmeal: Oats have the highest proportion of soluble fiber compared to any other grain.[66] Choose unsweetened plain oatmeal and add a small amount of honey or maple syrup.

Be aware: Your supermarket will carry a wide variety of breakfast cereal and oatmeal. Look for products that are low in sugar and that contain 100% whole grains. Be aware of marketing techniques and misleading nutritional claims on the packaging. The best choices are products that have a fiber content of at least 3 grams/100 calories, and a sugar content no higher than 10 grams/100 calories.

Canada's Food Guide recommends that at least half of all grain choices be whole grain foods. However, we recommend even higher levels. After researching the benefits of high fiber–low glycemic index foods, we recommend that you aim to eliminate refined grains from your diet entirely. Whole grain pasta, brown rice, and barley are readily available in all supermarkets, so it is merely a question of changing your habits. Grains and grain-like plant foods such as quinoa, bulgur, and wheat berries can be found in bulk food stores or health food stores. They are easy to make and will add variety to your diet. Consult our handy grain table on page 103 for simple cooking instructions.

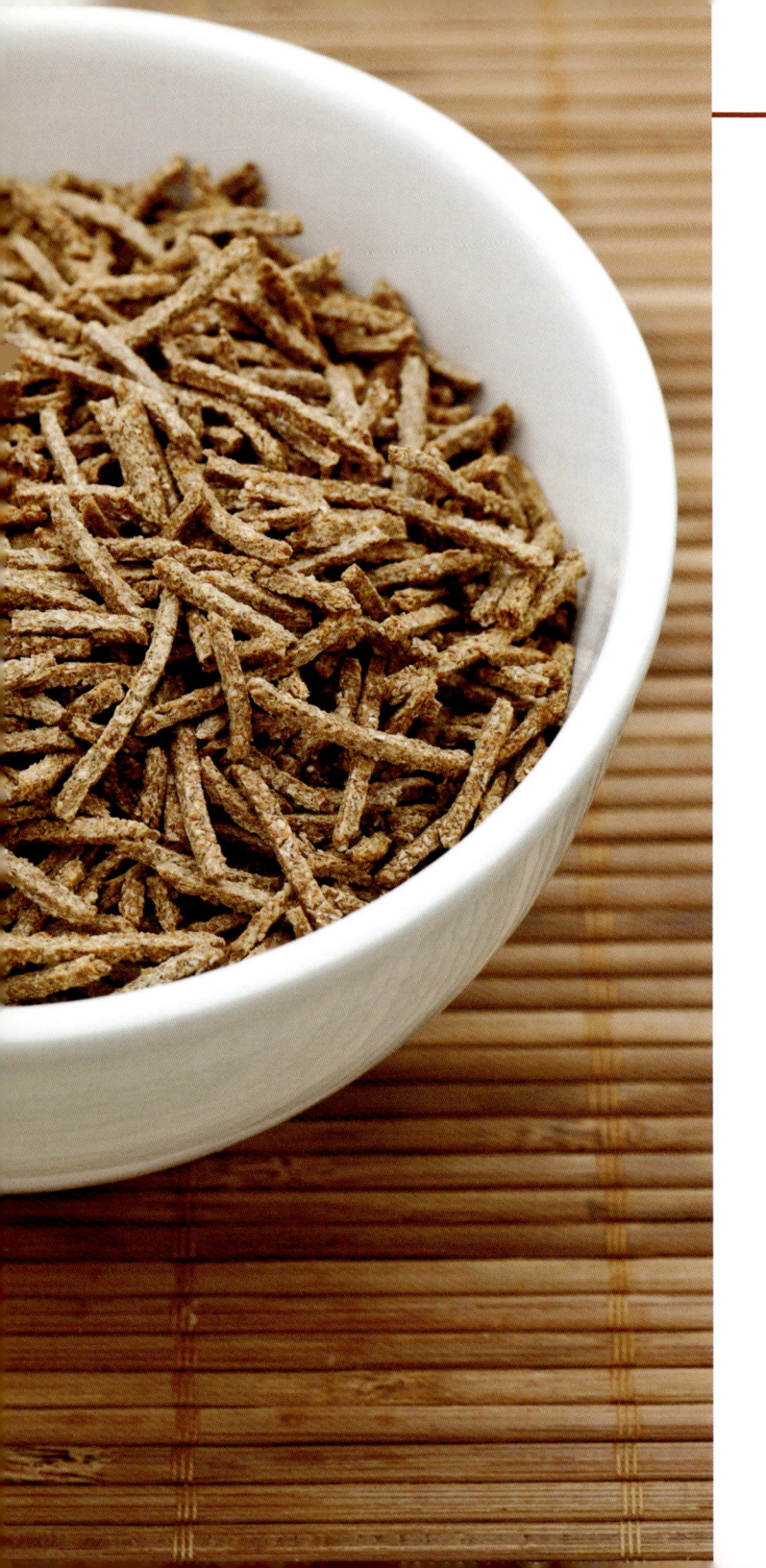

💡 Tips

- Choose steel-cut oatmeal or quick cooking oatmeal over instant oatmeal for a healthier option. Precook oatmeal and store it in the refrigerator for 2-3 days. Reheat for a quick breakfast.
- Mix different types of bran cereal for variety.
- Choose whole grain, whole wheat, flax seed, rye, or pumpernickel bread over white bread.
- Use barley or brown rice instead of white rice in stir-fry recipes.

🍽 Meal ideas

- Enjoy a bowl of bran cereal or oatmeal topped with berries or dried apricots. Add 1 tbsp of ground flax seed and 1 tbsp of wheat germ for a breakfast packed with eye nutrients.
- Top low-fat yogurt or ricotta cheese with bran cereal and fresh fruit for a tasty parfait.

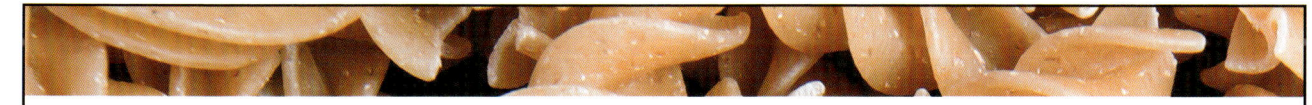

Whole Grains

Grain/Legume	Cooking Method
Whole wheat pasta	4 parts water : 1 part pasta Add to boiling water. Uncover, cook until al dente.
Brown rice	2 parts water : 1 part rice Bring water and rice to a boil. Cover and simmer for between 30-45 minutes. Cooking time may vary.
Barley (pearl)	2.5 parts water : 1 part barley Add to boiling water. Partially cover, simmer for 30-40 minutes or until water is absorbed.
Quinoa	2 parts water : 1 part quinoa Rinse very well. Add to boiling water. Partially cover and simmer for 15-18 minutes or until water is absorbed.
Wheat berries	3 parts water : 1 part wheat berries Bring water and wheat berries to a boil. Partially cover and simmer for about 1 hour or until water is absorbed.
Bulgur	2 parts water : 1 part bulgur Add to boiling water. Cover and simmer for 7-12 minutes or until water has been absorbed.

Eyefoods   Chapter 3

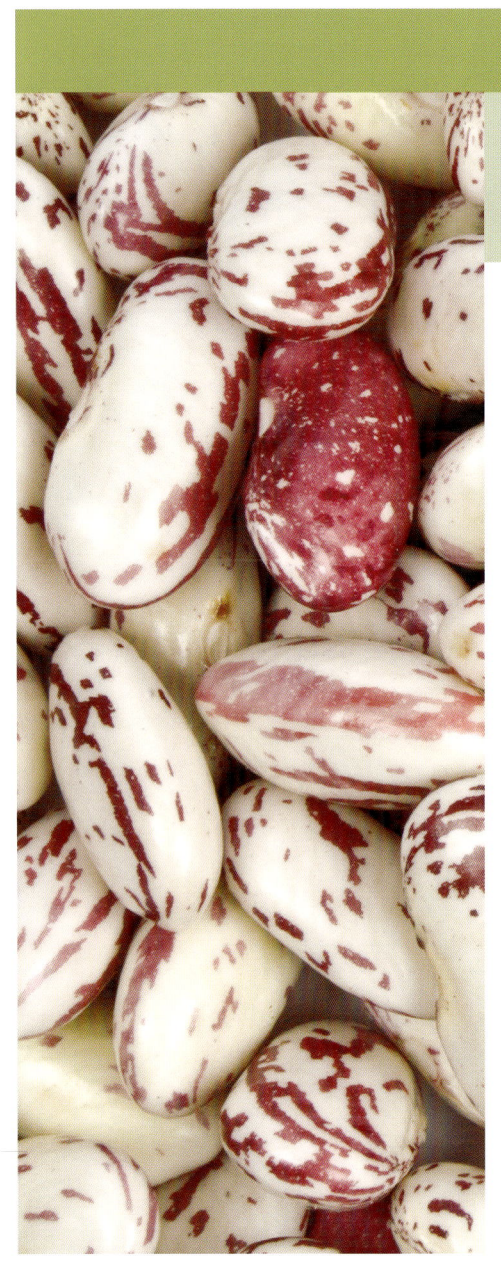

Beans and Lentils

Black beans, Romano beans, red kidney beans, soybeans (edamame), white beans, chick peas, green, black, and red lentils

Eye nutrients:
Fiber, omega-3 fatty acids (ALA), zinc

Weekly target:
Beans or lentils: ½ cup 4 times per week
Edamame (soybeans): ½ cup 2 times per week

Overview:
Because cardiovascular disease and age-related macular degeneration share many common risk factors, a heart friendly diet is also an eye-friendly diet. Beans and lentils are a great source of fiber and protein and contain a minimal amount of fat, so they play an important role in a diet that is ideal for both the heart and the eyes. Many different cultures use beans and lentils in their cuisine. East-Indian cuisine features lentils, Mediterranean cuisine includes Romano and white beans, Mexican cuisine relies on red kidney and black beans, and Asian cuisine makes good use of soybeans. Even the typical North American diet includes beans, mainly the navy beans found in baked beans.

Part 2   The Details

How to buy: Beans are available in many different forms. The easiest way to include beans in your diet is to buy them canned. However, canned beans tend to have a high sodium content, so we recommend rinsing canned beans thoroughly.

Top Eyefoods:
Romano beans, black beans, soybeans (edamame)

Romano beans and black beans: These are top eyefoods because they are very high in fiber and contain significant amounts of zinc.

Soybeans (edamame): These score highly as an eyefood due to their high content of omega-3 fatty acids (ALA). They are available in the pod or shelled and can be found in the freezer section of your grocery store.

💡 Tips

- Rinse canned beans well in a colander under running water to get rid of excess sodium.
- Add canned beans to soups, stews, or sautéed dishes.
- Use green lentils instead of rice as a side dish for fish.
- Add shelled soybeans to stir-fries, soups, or salads.
- Drink plenty of water to avoid the gassy effects of eating beans.

🍽 Meal ideas

- Make a colorful bean salad with canned beans, orange peppers, sun-dried tomatoes and green onions.
- Enjoy hummus (chick pea spread) as a sandwich filler or dip.
- Try soybeans in the pod (edamame) as an appetizer: sprinkle with salt and sesame seeds and eat with your fingers. Avoid eating the pod, as it is very tough.
- Toss cooked white beans or chick peas with olive oil and your favorite mix of spices. (Start with cumin, curry, and coriander.) Roast in a 400 °F (200 °C) oven for 40 minutes for a crunchy snack.

Eyefoods   Chapter 3

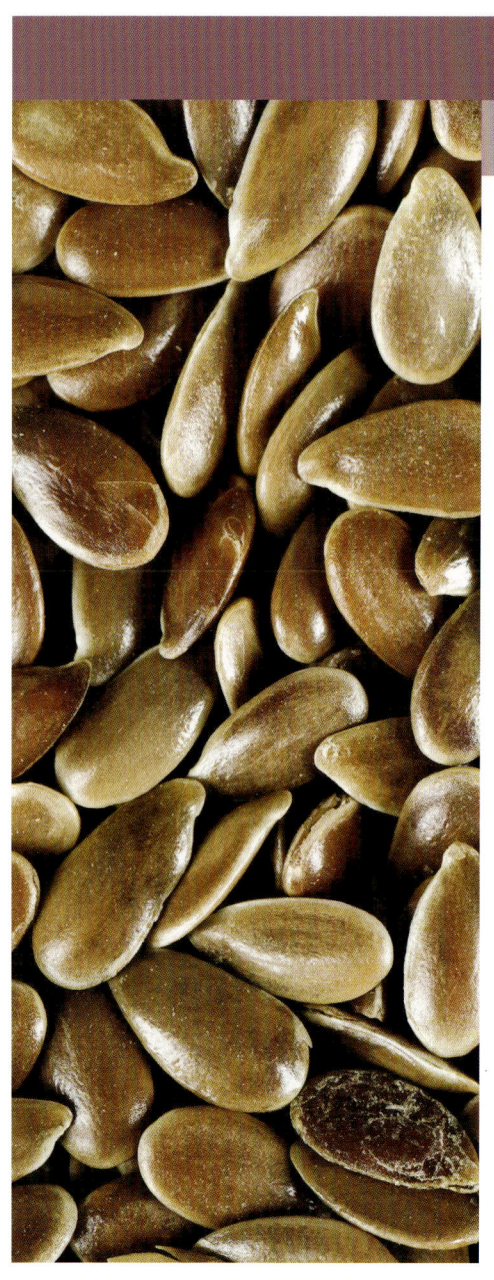

Flax Seed

Ground flax seed, flax seed oil

Eye nutrients:
Omega-3 fatty acids (ALA), fiber, vitamin E, zinc

Weekly target:
1 tablespoon ground flax seed or wheat germ per day

Overview:
With significant amounts of plant-derived omega-3 fatty acids (ALA), fiber, vitamin E and zinc, ground flax seed and flax seed oil are essential eyefoods. Flax seed has a particular benefit for people who have dry-eye syndrome. Studies have shown that daily consumption of flax seed oil reduces symptoms of dry eye syndrome in people with Sjogren's syndrome.[67]

Even though flax seed contains a significant amount of omega-3 fatty acids (ALA), flax seed should be consumed in addition to fish, not as a substitute for it. Our bodies do convert ALA to DHA and EPA (the omega-3 fatty acids abundant in fish), but not very efficiently. There are many different kinds of omega-3 fatty acids. The main ones used by our bodies are DHA and EPA, found in fish.

Part 2   The Details

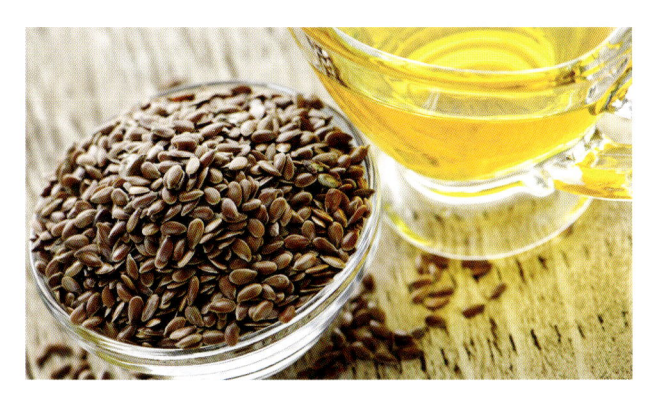

💡 Tips

- Grind your flax seed! Our bodies cannot break down the outer coating of the whole seed. A coffee grinder will work well for this.
- Whole flax is stable at room temperature and will remain fresh for several months.
- Once opened, store flax seed oil in the refrigerator and use within six weeks.

🍽 Meal ideas

- Add ground flax seed to bran cereal or oatmeal.
- Mix ground flax seed into carrot muffin batter to make a tasty eyefood treat.

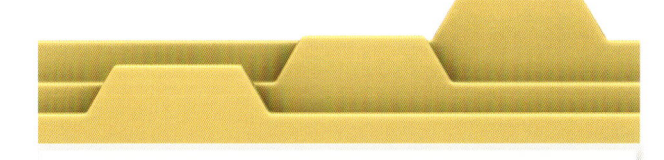

QUICK AND EASY RECIPE

Eyefoods Smoothie with Flax Seed

½ cup diced cantaloupe
½ cup strawberries
½ mango
½ cup unsweetened orange juice
2 tbsp ground flax seed

Cut cantaloupe and mango in cubes and place in a blender. Add strawberries, orange juice, and flax seed. Blend on high until mixture is a smooth consistency. Best enjoyed immediately.

Makes 2 smoothies.

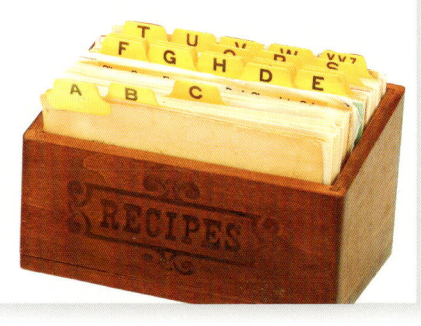

Eyefoods   Chapter 3

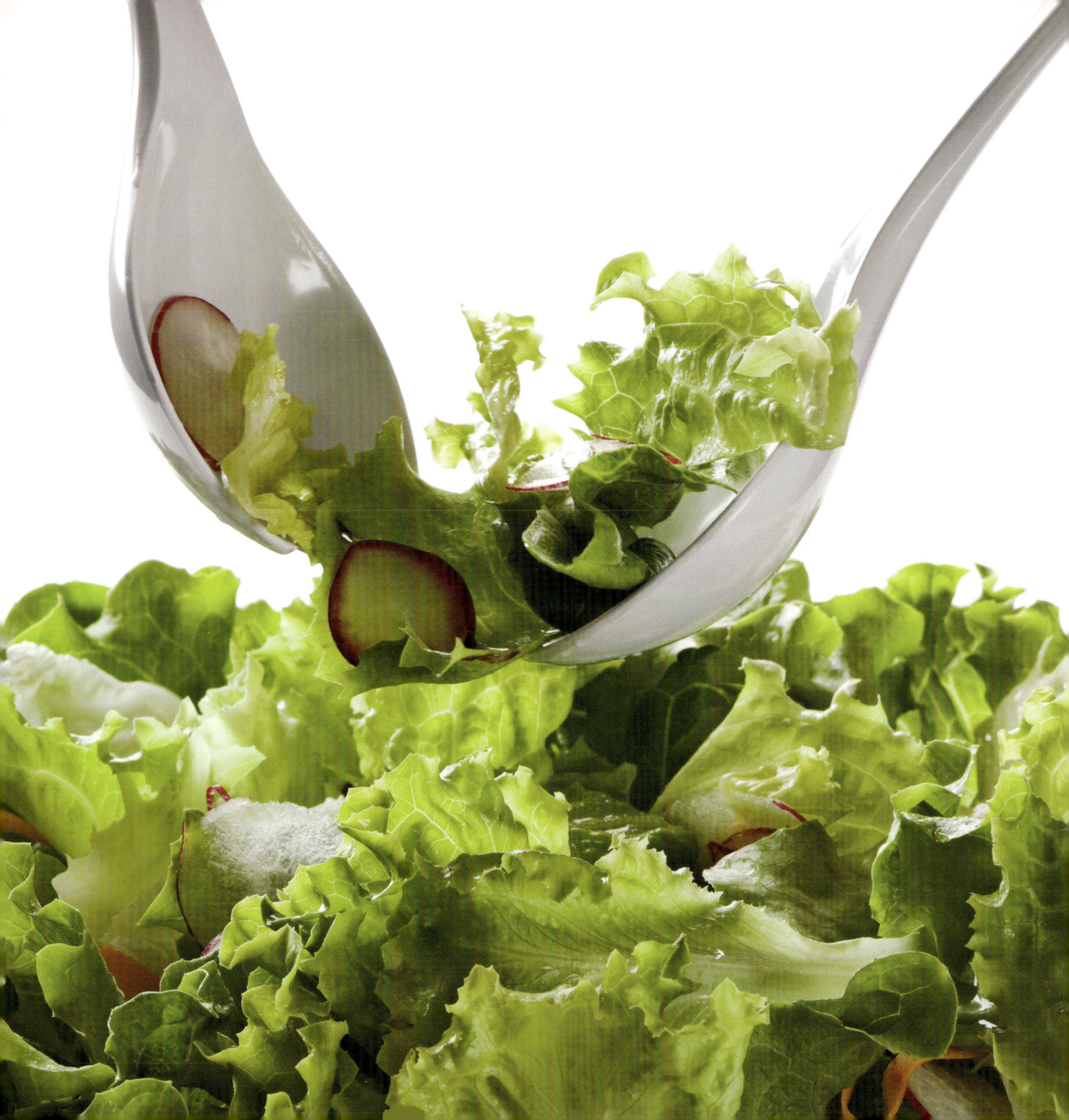

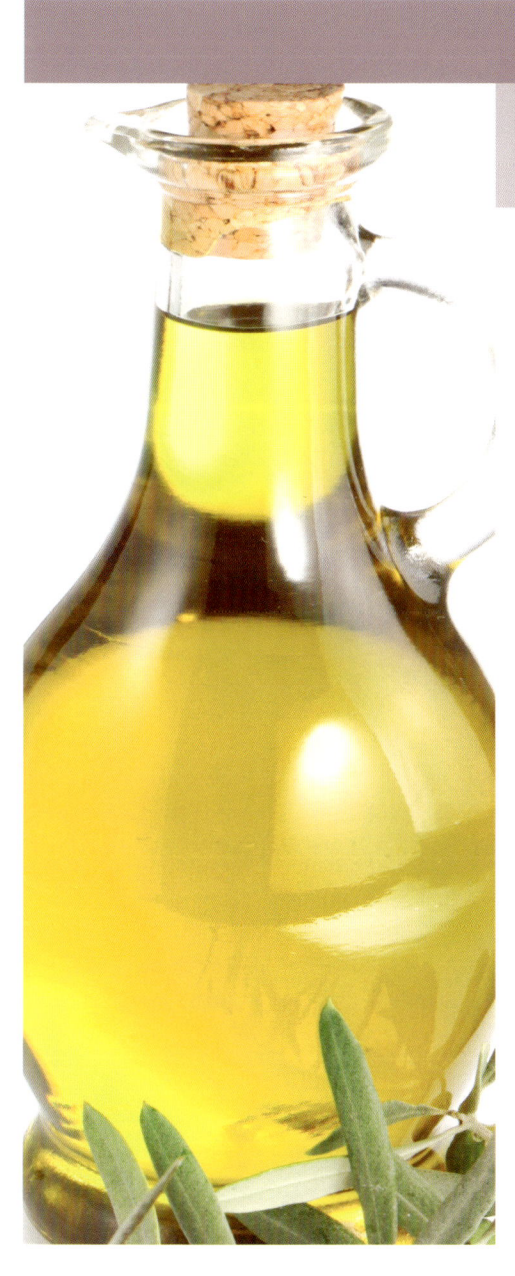

Oil

Canola oil, extra virgin olive oil, flax seed oil, walnut oil

Eye nutrients:
Omega-3 fatty acids, vitamin E

Weekly target:
2 tbsp canola or olive oil per day

Overview:
Canola oil and extra virgin olive oil are included as eyefoods because they are healthful monounsaturated fats that contain vitamin E and ALA. Flax seed oil contains higher levels of omega-3 fatty acids and vitamin E. Walnut oil is a nice occasional treat in a delicate salad. Grape seed oil has a high burning point, making it excellent to use in a stir-fry. Remember that fat from any source is calorie-dense, so you should eat only a minimal amount to avoid an expanding waistline.

Top Eyefoods: Extra virgin olive oil, canola oil

Olive oil: A monounsaturated fat and a good source of vitamin E.

Canola oil: A monounsaturated fat and a good source of vitamin E and ALA.

> **Canada's Food Guide recommends:**
> - Include a small amount of unsaturated fat (2-3 tbsp or 30-45 mL) each day. This includes cooking oils, dressings, margarine, and mayonnaise.
> - Use vegetable oils such as olive oil, canola oil, or soybean oil.
> - Limit butter, lard, hard margarine, and shortening.

💡 Tips

- Use canola oil or olive oil instead of butter as often as you can.
- Choose canola oil or extra virgin olive oil. It is the first-pressed olive oil and has the best flavor and health benefits.
- Store flax seed oil and walnut oil in the refrigerator to extend their shelf life.
- Mix equal parts extra virgin olive oil and canola oil in a canister or jar. Use this as your cooking oil or for dressings and marinades.
- All oils contain over 100 calories per tablespoon, so consume in small quantities.

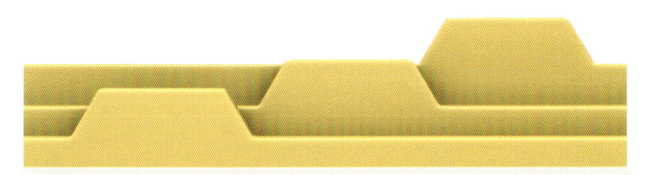

QUICK AND EASY RECIPE

Eyefoods Basic Salad Dressing

¼ cup olive oil
¼ cup canola oil
3 tbsp apple cider vinegar
1 tbsp lemon juice
1 tbsp Dijon mustard
1 tbsp maple syrup
Sea salt and black pepper to taste

Whisk together all ingredients. Transfer to a glass jar and store in the refrigerator for up to two weeks.

Makes ¾ cup.

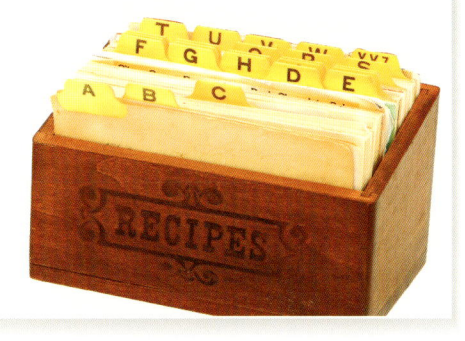

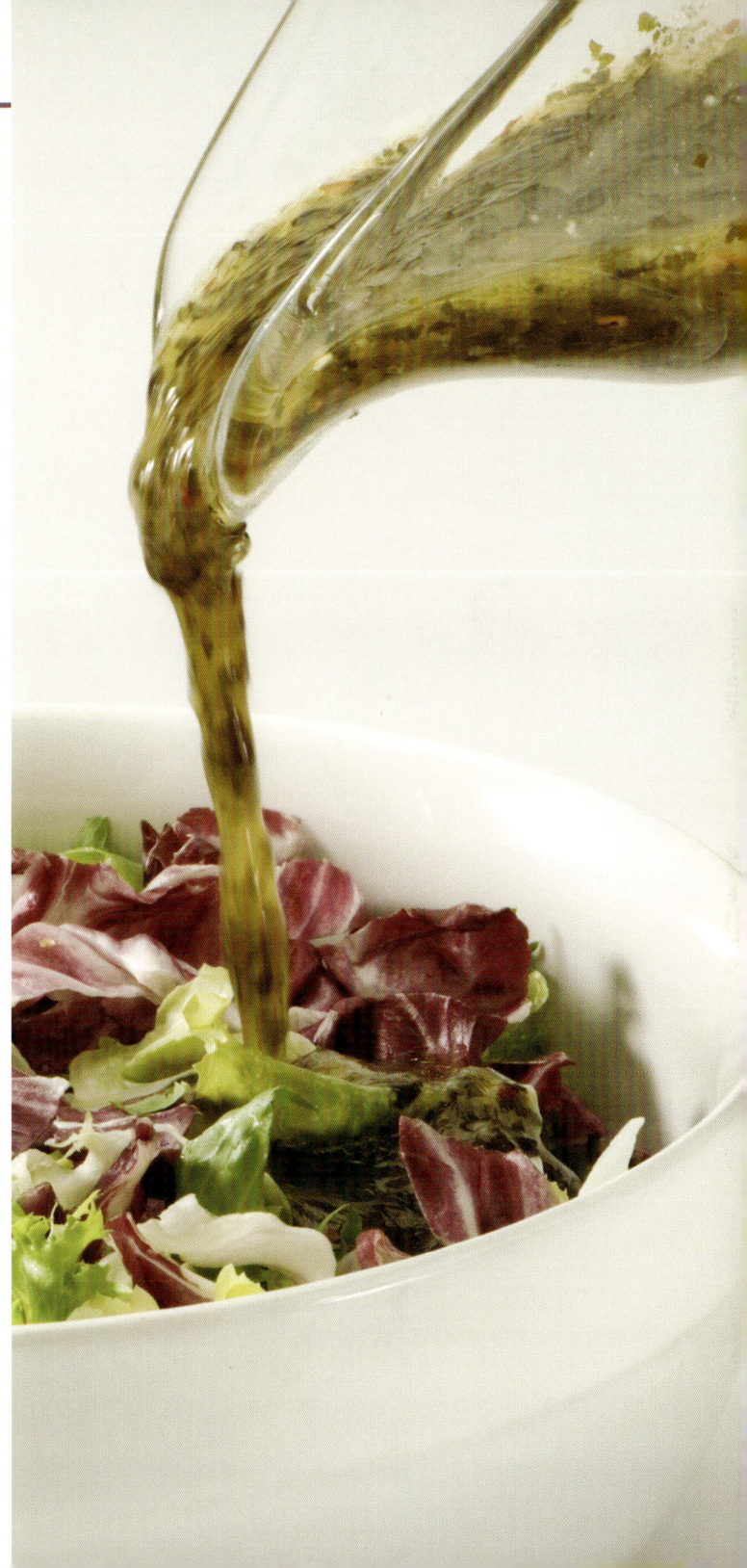

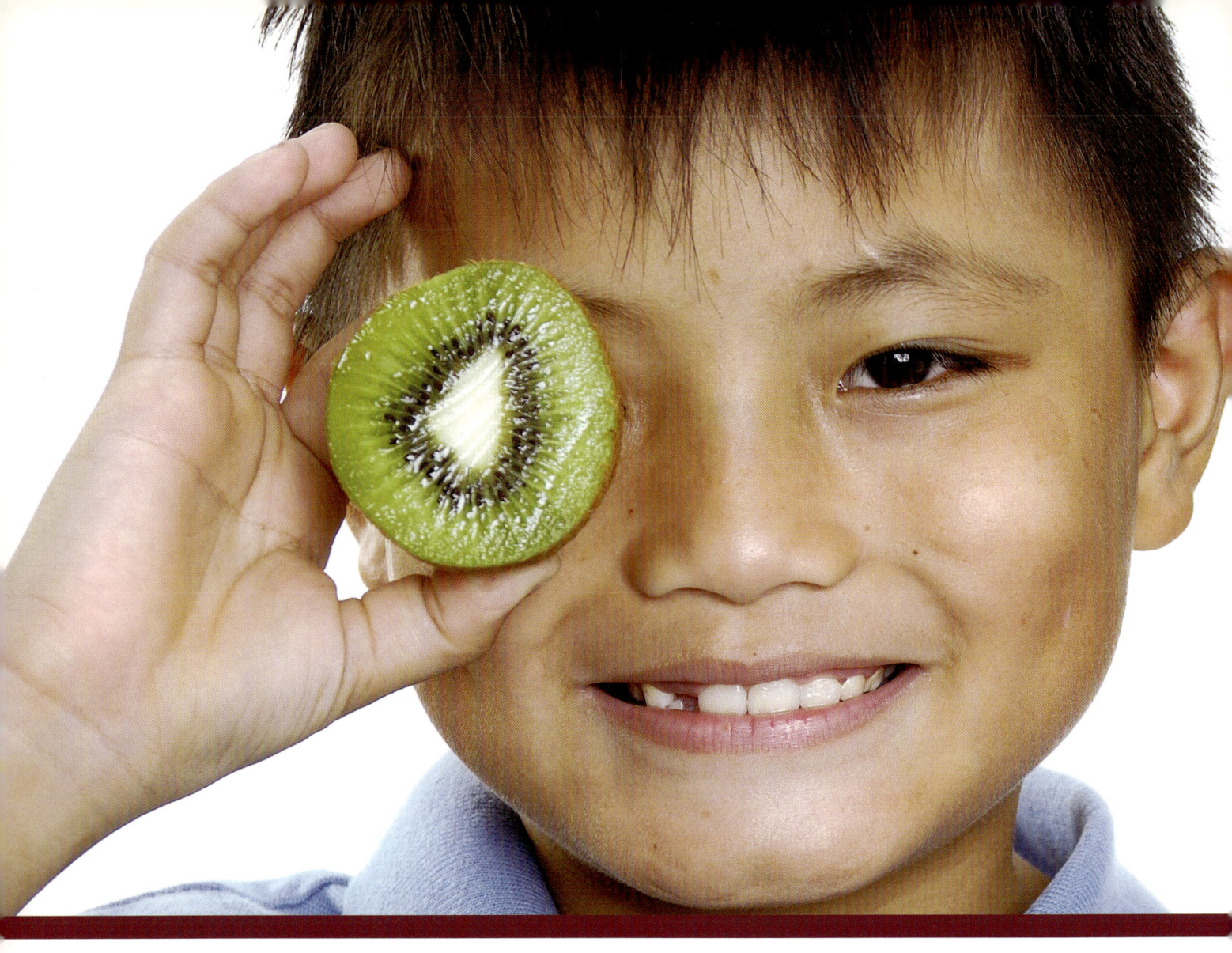

Eating eyefoods will lead you down the path to better eye health. Living a healthy lifestyle as well will have a great impact on the prevention of eye disease. The eyefoods lifestyle recommendations will help you to improve your eye health and general well-being.

Chapter 4
Lifestyle and General Health

We all know that proper nutrition is essential to our well-being. In addition to promoting long-term general health, developing good eating habits will nourish your eyes. The previous chapters made recommendations for your eyes with respect to nutrition. But other parts of your lifestyle will also directly affect the health of your eyes. For instance, you may be aware that smoking increases the risk for AMD, but did you know that regular exercise can help prevent certain eye diseases?

The benefits of leading a healthy lifestyle are numerous. When you make healthy lifestyle choices, you are taking control of your overall physical health. You will also notice that you feel better in other ways: you will have the energy and vitality you need to lead a happy and fulfilling life. Our lifestyle recommendations for preventing eye disease will also promote long-term general health.

Our patients ask us on a daily basis how they can protect their vision. This chapter will explain how your lifestyle decisions can benefit your eyes and your everyday life.

UV and Blue Light Exposure

The sun and certain types of lamps (such as those used in tanning beds) emit ultraviolet radiation. Researchers have found that overexposure to UV light may cause cataracts, age-related macular degeneration, skin cancer, sunburns, and premature aging of the skin. Health Canada recommends avoiding overexposure to UV light and tanning beds, wearing sunglasses, and using sunscreen to protect against the harmful effects of UV light.[68]

Blue light (short wavelength visible light) causes oxidative stress to the retina. This particularly affects people with less of the macular pigments lutein and zeaxanthin. People with light-colored irides, people with AMD, and people with a genetic predisposition to AMD are more susceptible to the harmful effects of blue light.[69]

UV light, blue light, and eye disease:
A large European study showed a significant relationship between blue light and new blood vessel growth in the retina in patients with early AMD and low levels of antioxidants. These findings reinforce the theory that diet and lifestyle are both important in the prevention of eye disease. Another significant study found that sunlight exposure in young adult life is associated with the development of early AMD.[70]

UV light and general health:
Overexposure to UV light may cause skin cancer, sunburn, and premature aging of the skin.

Be aware:
Babies, children, and young adults have more transparent lenses in their eyes and more sensitive skin on their bodies. As a result, they are at a greater risk of experiencing the adverse effects of overexposure to UV light. The effects of overexposure to UV light at a younger age may not show up until later in life.[71]

At 20 years of age, the average person has received 80% of their life's UV exposure. This is why it is critical to effectively protect our children's eyes from the sun, beginning from their birth and continuing throughout their childhood.

Part 2   The Details

UV Exposure

Sunglasses

When it comes to choosing sunglasses, the options are endless. The choices can be confusing if you do not have some important background information. Not all lenses are equal in terms of UV- and blue light protection. The optical quality of the lens, the level of protection, and the longevity of such protection vary greatly. Here are a few helpful tips.

Visible light and UV light:
The light spectrum is categorized by wavelength. If the light is in the visible spectrum, the wavelengths will determine its color. If it is in the ultraviolet range, these wavelengths determine its UV category (A, B or C).

Blue wavelength light:
Blue wavelength light can damage the retina, leading to AMD and blurring of vision.

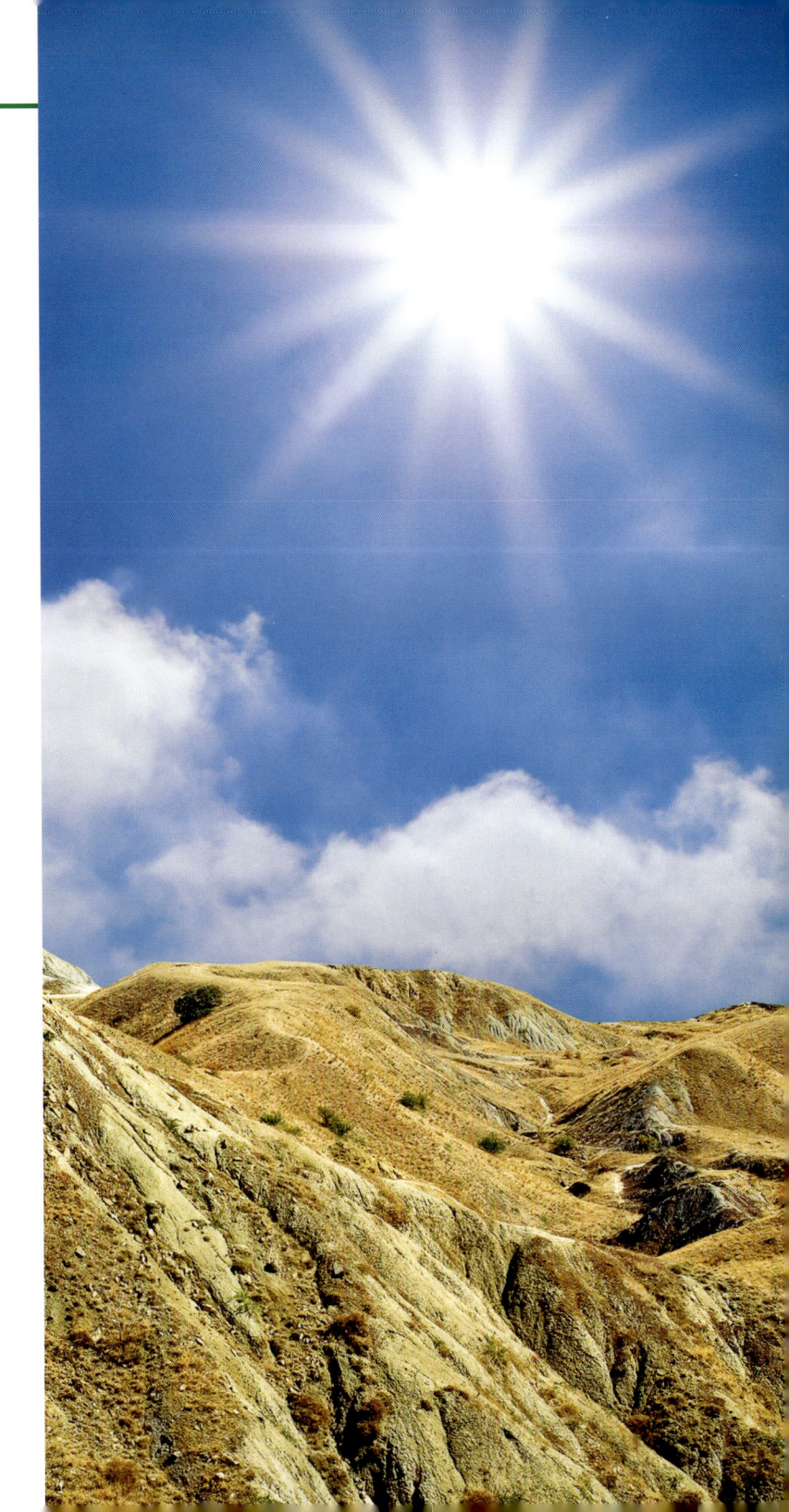

Types of glare:
Direct glare is the bright sunlight that comes from the sun above and its reflection below. *Reflected glare* is produced by flat, smooth, and shiny surfaces, like a car windshield, the surface of a lake, or the puddles on the road. *Bounce-back glare* reaches you from your side and from behind.

The difference between a high quality pair of sunglasses and a low quality pair of sunglasses is measured by the UV protection they give and by the way they filter blue light. The gold standard in sunglasses for UV protection has been UV 400, which will protect against UV categories A, B, and C. (It may help to remember that UV**A** relates to aging, UV**B** to burning, and UV**C** to cancer.)

However, scientists have recently found that visible blue light also has damaging effects on the eyes, so optimal sun protection includes a selective blue filter.[72] The once-popular "Blue Blocker" lens blocked all blue rays of light, though it also changed the quality of the colors seen through the glasses.

Lens features

1. The color, or tint, of the sunglass lens does not affect its UV- and blue light protection. In fact, you can get a clear UV 400 coating on your lenses. Cheaply made UV 400 sunglasses will have a spray-on coating that will wear off with cleaning, giving you a false sense of security, and not all brands of lenses will have blue light filters. A quality pair of sunglasses will filter blue light as well as UV light. While still absorbing the damaging energy of blue light, these glasses will allow you to see colors normally.
2. A mirror on the front of your lenses will reflect most of the direct glare, essentially "squinting" so you don't have to.
3. A polarized filter embedded in your sunglasses will eliminate reflected glare from the road, water, windshields, and other flat shiny

Part 2   The Details

surfaces. With polarized lenses, you can see below the water's surface, so they are great for fishing.
4. A back surface anti-reflective coating will prevent light from bouncing off the back of the lens and into your eyes. This feature reduces glare.
5. A photochromic lens will adjust to lighting conditions, getting darker as the light gets brighter. A photochromic lens is activated by UV rays, so the lens will not change as much when you are inside a car.
6. Excellent quality plastic lenses will be impact-resistant, light-weight, and treated with an anti-scratch coating. They will have high-quality optics, giving you sharper vision.
7. Glass lenses are heavier, more resistant to scratching, and provide crisp optics. As they are not impact-resistant and may shatter, they are not well suited for sports use.
8. You can choose the color of the tint of your sunglasses depending on your visual needs, the intended use for the sunglasses, and your personal preference. Brown-colored tints increase contrast, while grey-colored tints do not change color perception.
9. Specialized tints are available for different sports and activities. You can get lenses that maximize your vision for tennis, golf, hunting, and fishing, just to name a few.

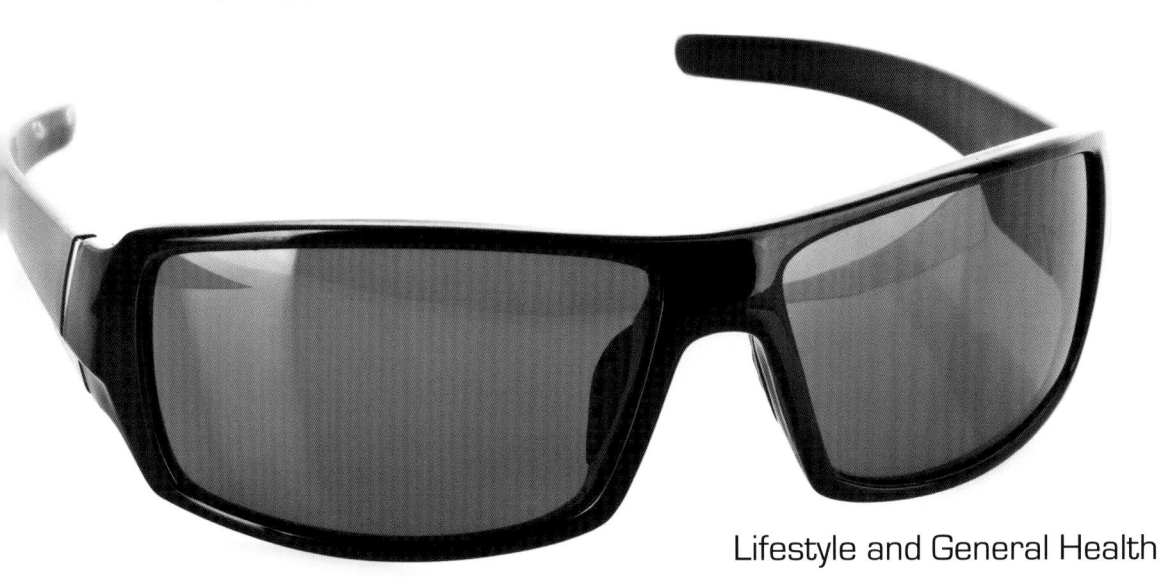

Lifestyle and General Health   Chapter 4

Sunglass Frames

1. When choosing a sunglass frame, the most important thing to consider is its fit. The frame should fit close to your eyes and face to reduce the entry of bounce-back glare. The frame has to be big enough to provide appropriate coverage and protection for your eyes.
2. Most quality sunglasses will be available with your own prescription, so you don't have to put up with wearing two pairs of glasses on top of each other.
3. Clip-on sunglasses are available for most prescription glasses. Although these are an acceptable compromise, they add to the weight of your glasses, causing them to slip down your nose. Also, there will be internal reflection between the two sets of lenses that decreases the quality of your vision. With frequent use, the clip may cause paint to chip off your frame.
4. If you choose the clip-on or a photochromic lens, you should be aware that light will still reach you from around the frame. This is because regular eye glasses are usually smaller and flatter than sunglasses, and do not fit as close to your face.

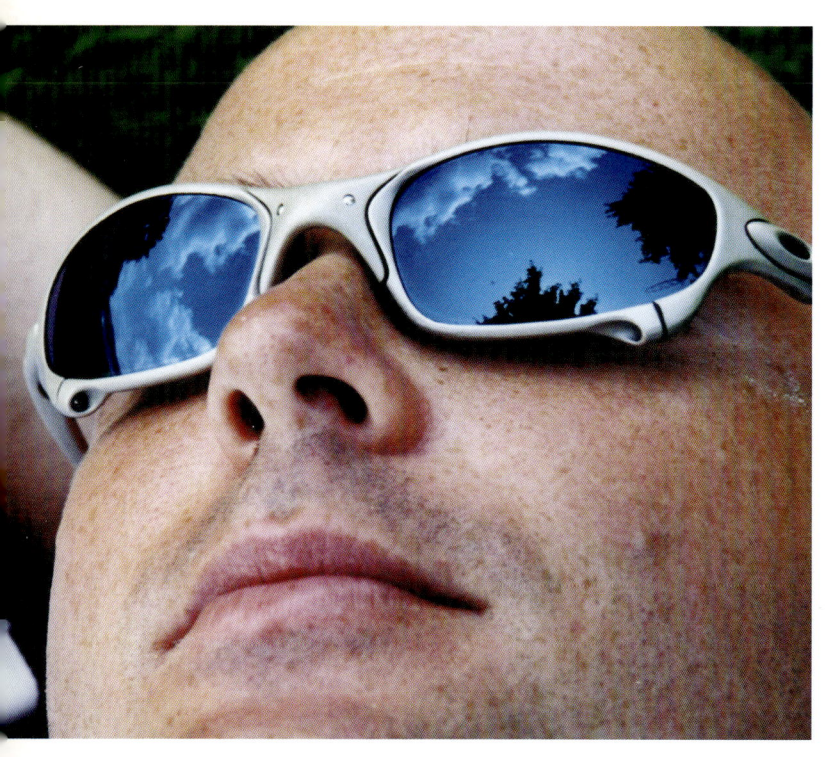

Part 2   The Details

IN SUMMARY

Have a professional help you to choose your sunglasses.

Because there are many options available, you will find it helpful to consult an expert when you are trying to choose which sunglasses will be best suited to your needs. Do some research ahead of time so you have a good idea about your preferences, and then see your optician or optometrist for help. He or she may be able to recommend the perfect pair for you.

The best way to see clearly and distortion-free is to have a pair of polarized prescription sunglasses.

These will eliminate 100% of UV light, filter blue light, reduce glare, and stay dark in your car when you are driving.

Lifestyle and General Health   Chapter 4

Smoking

The dangerous effects of smoking have long been proven. Most people are well aware that smoking greatly increases the risk of cancer and heart disease, but other parts of the body are affected by smoking as well. Scientific studies show that smoking is the most important modifiable risk factor in age-related macular degeneration.[73]

Smoking and eye disease:
Smoking is the number one modifiable risk factor in AMD prevention. Scientists have found that, compared to people who have never smoked, current smokers are 45% more likely to develop early AMD or AMD progression over 15 years.[74]

Smoking and general health:
Research shows there to be a direct link between smoking and the development of cancer and heart disease.

Be aware:
A study has found that current smokers and recent ex-smokers who took high dose beta-carotene supplements had an increased risk for developing lung cancer. People who smoke are advised not to take supplements that contain beta-carotene, although beta-carotene found in food is considered safe.[75] Most manufacturers of eye vitamins have introduced products without beta-carotene or have taken beta-carotene out of their formulations. AREDS-2 is currently studying formulations without beta-carotene.

Health Canada recommends:
- Visit www.hc-sc.gc.ca/hc-ps/tobac-tabac/quit-cessser/now-maintenant/index-eng.php for help with quitting smoking.[76]

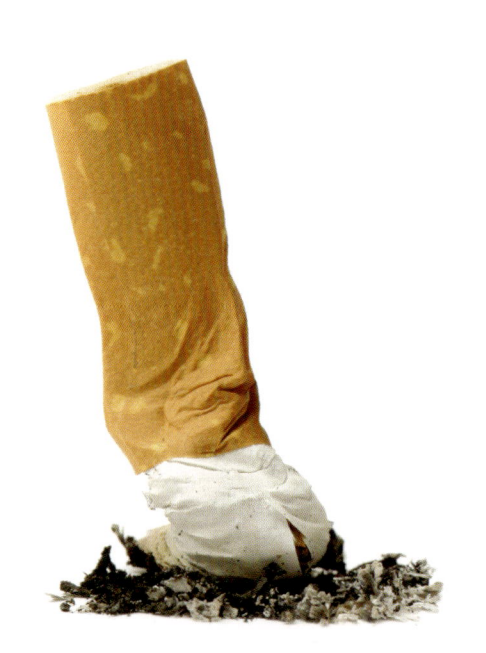

Part 2   The Details

Body Mass Index (BMI) and Waist Circumference:

Health Canada recommends maintaining a healthy body weight to help prevent chronic disease and improve your general health. The World Health Organization (WHO) and Health Canada recognize body mass index (BMI) and waist circumference as the two measurements used by professionals to help determine a person's risk for developing diseases associated with being overweight. (Note that these tools do not apply to children under the age of 18 or to pregnant or lactating women).[77]

BMI:
BMI is a ratio of weight to height. You can calculate your BMI by consulting an online BMI table or by using the formula BMI = weight (kg)/height (m)^2. A normal BMI is between 18.5 and 24.9. A BMI over 25 is in the overweight category, and a BMI over 30 is in the obese category. People in the overweight or obese categories have a higher risk of developing health problems.[78]

Waist circumference:
Waist circumference is an indicator of abdominal obesity and pertains to an apple-shaped body. Health Canada recognizes that men with a waist circumference greater than 40 inches and women with a waist circumference greater than 35 inches have an increased risk of developing certain chronic health conditions.[79]

BMI, waist circumference, and eye disease:
An above-normal BMI may be associated with an increased risk of age-related macular degeneration. A larger waist circumference or waist-to-hip ratio may increase the likelihood of the progression of AMD.[80]

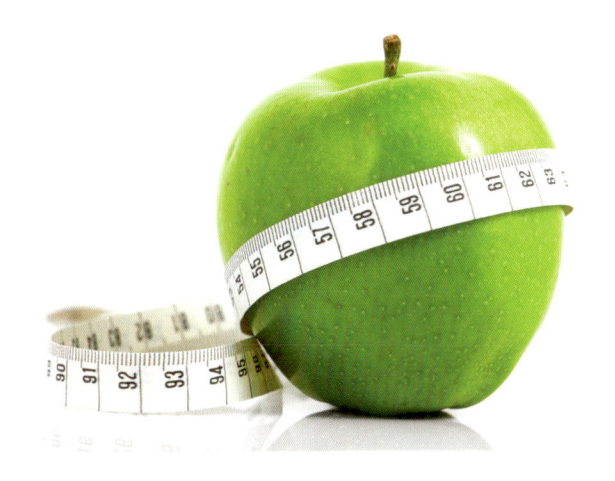

Lifestyle and General Health   Chapter 4

Physical Activity

Physical activity is essential for a healthy lifestyle. We are all aware of the long-term health benefits of exercise and physical activity, but making physical activity a regular part of your life will help you feel younger, stronger, and more energetic right now.

Exercise daily:
Go for a walk or enjoy the scenery on a bike ride. Physical activity stimulates blood circulation, nourishing and detoxifying your cells. Exercise benefits your heart and arteries, and therefore your eyes and vision.

Physical activity and eye disease:
We recommend regular physical activity as part of an eye-friendly lifestyle. Scientists believe that exercising at least three times per week can slow the progression of age-related macular degeneration.[81]

Physical activity and general health:
Increased physical activity can decrease the risk of cardiovascular disease and stroke. Other health benefits of regular physical activity include weight control, stronger muscles and bones, reduced stress, and increased energy and vitality.[82]

> **The Public Health Agency of Canada recommends:**
> - **Adults:** 2.5 hours of moderate to vigorous intensity physical activity per week
> - **Children and youth:** 60 minutes of moderate to vigorous intensity physical activity per day
> - If you have any health concerns, consult your physician before starting any new exercise program.

Age-Related Macular Degeneration (AMD) and Cardiovascular Disease

Current scientific studies show a relationship between AMD and cardiovascular disease. AMD and cardiovascular disease share many of the same risk factors, including age, smoking, antioxidant levels, physical activity, BMI, and waist circumference.

Part 2   The Details

In 2006 a study regarding the relationship between cardiovascular disease and AMD found that patients with AMD had a higher risk of stroke independent of other risk factors for stroke. Another study found that people with AMD between the ages of 49 and 75 had a greater long-term risk of having serious complications related to cardiovascular disease and stroke.[83]

Eye-friendly and heart-friendly lifestyles: Many similarities exist between eye-friendly and heart-friendly lifestyles, including getting good nutrition, engaging in physical activity, and not smoking. Recent scientific studies are starting to show a relationship between cardiovascular disease and AMD, but independently, the long-standing research for each of these diseases shows similar findings.

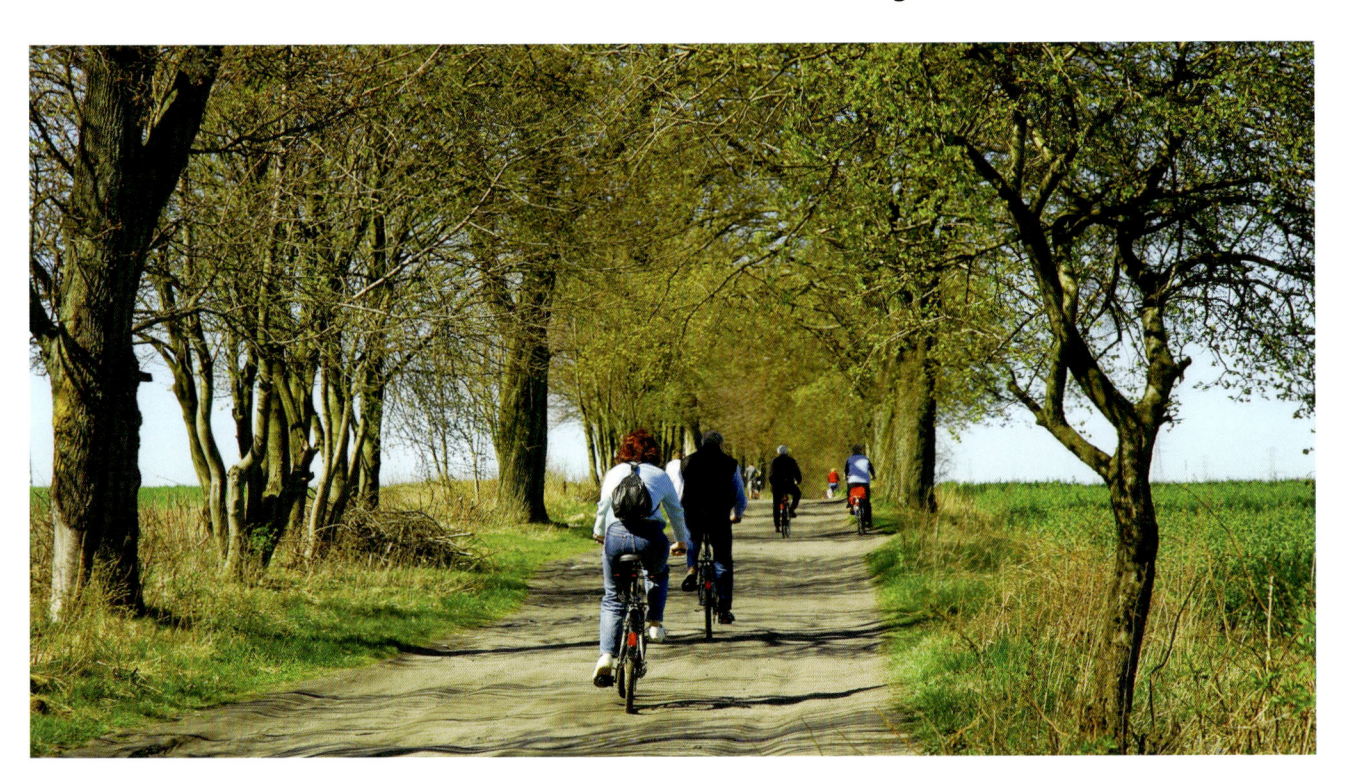

Healthy eyes, healthy heart, healthy body.

Lifestyle and General Health   Chapter 4

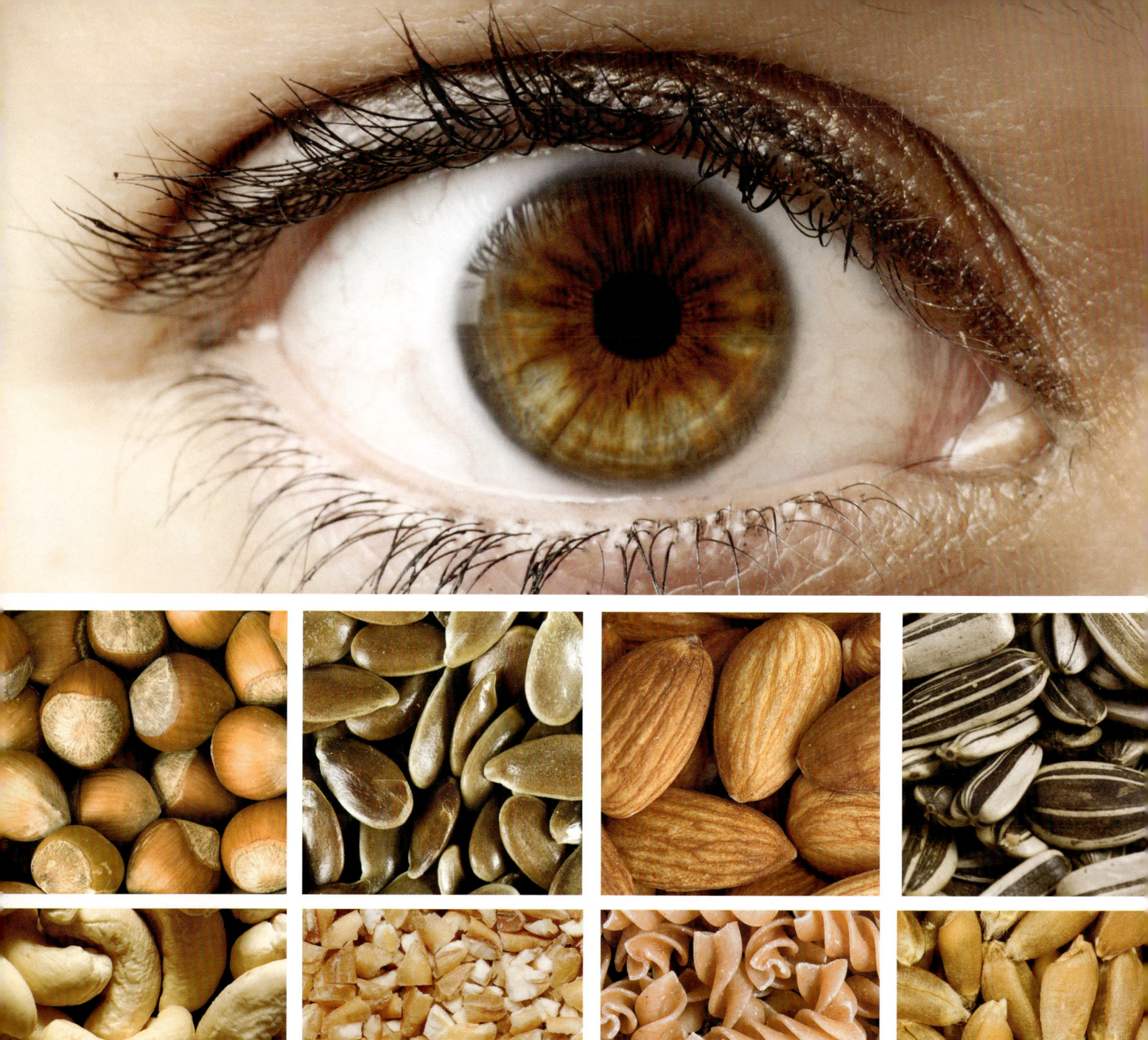

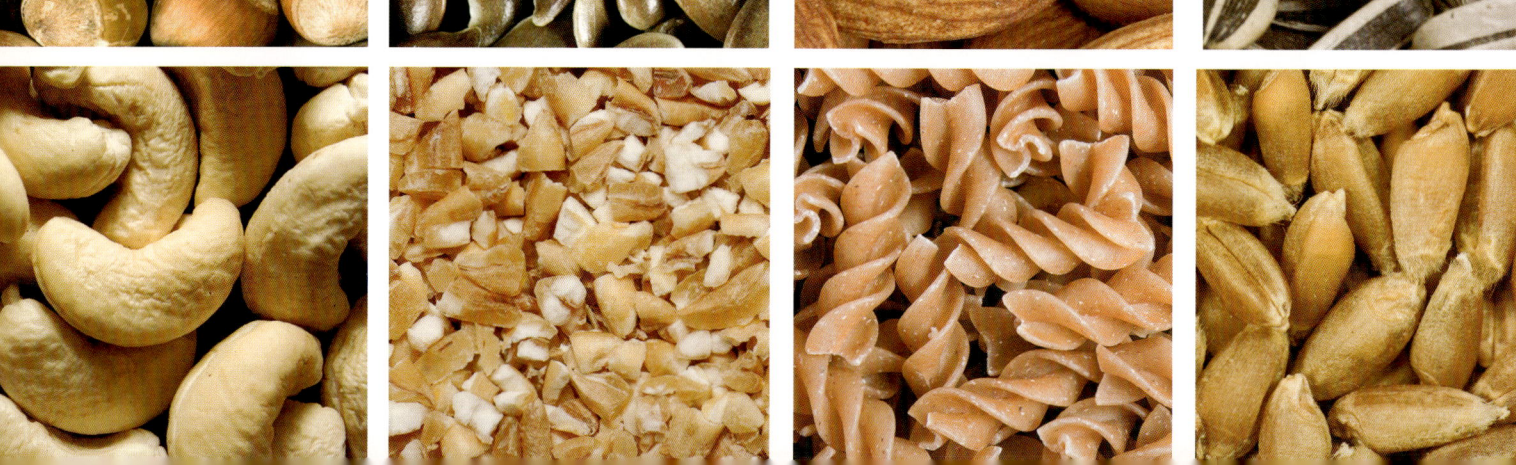

Part Three
The Plan

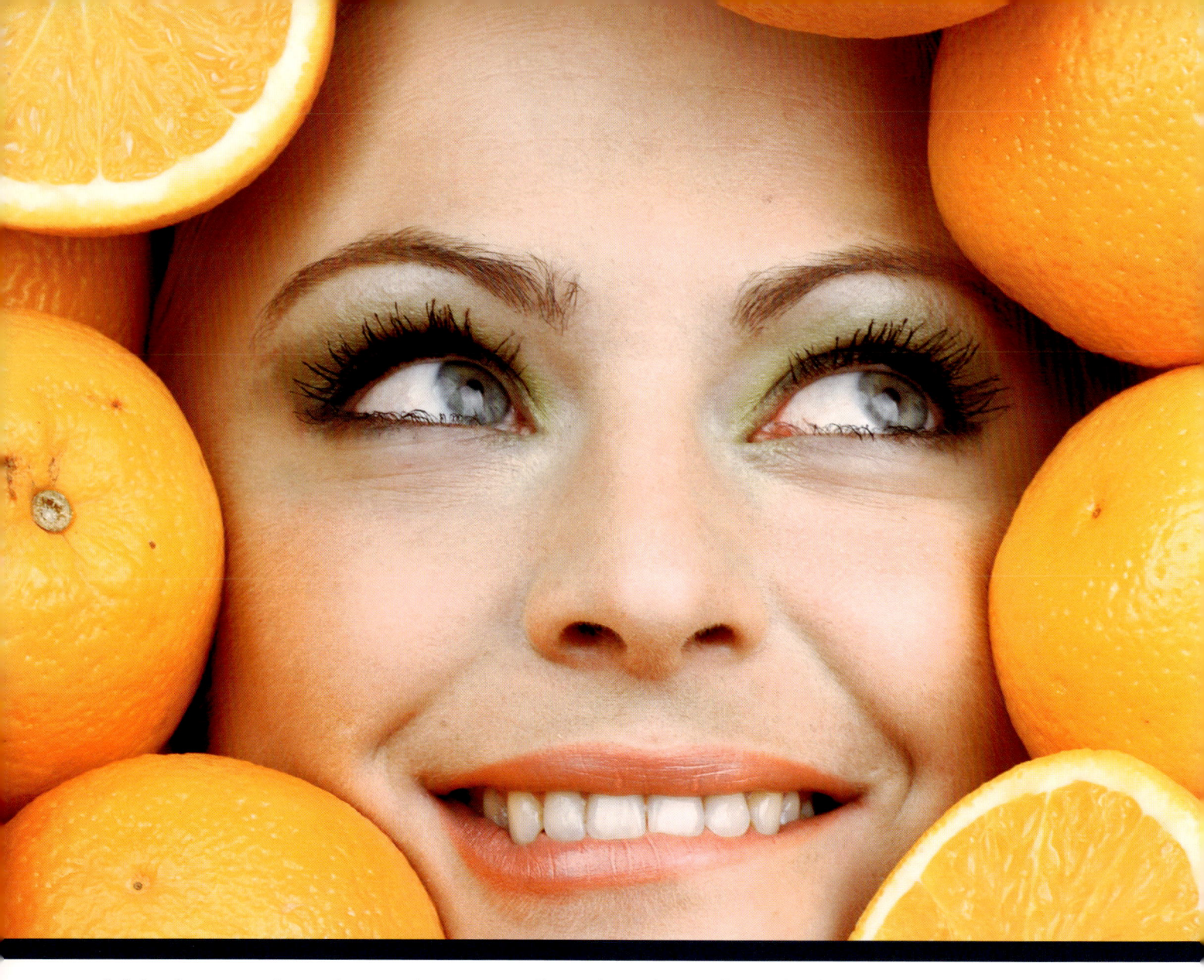

We have developed an eyefoods plan that is based on scientific research related to nutrition and eye health. The eyefoods plan will provide you with a simple way to integrate eyefoods and eyefoods lifestyle recommendations into your life.

Chapter 5
The Eyefoods Plan

In the previous chapters we discussed the food and lifestyle choices that can reduce your risk of developing age-related macular degeneration, cataracts, dry eye syndrome and eyelid disorders. We identified the nutrients that offer the greatest protection against eye disease, and we introduced eyefoods, the foods that are richest in these nutrients. In this chapter, we offer The eyefoods plan, a simple way to integrate eyefoods into your life.

The eyefoods plan outlines weekly targets for eyefoods, offers simple ways to identify serving sizes, and provides you with a plan to track your weekly eyefood consumption. The plan also provides guidelines on other lifestyle factors that are important to eye health, including eye supplements, sun protection, smoking, exercise, and weight management.

Following the eyefoods plan will help you to prevent eye disease and maintain a strong, healthy body. As we explained in the previous chapters, the eyefoods plan can also help you to reduce your risk of developing other chronic diseases. The eyefoods plan is a great way to complement a healthy diet and lifestyle.

In our modern world, there is a seemingly endless selection of health resources available to us, particularly in the media and on the Web. These diverse recommendations and reports can cause confusion. Sometimes, health topics reported in the media will conflict with recommendations that you may have received from your own health care provider. Be aware that not all published information on health is accurate. Health information should come from a reliable source that backs up its findings with accurate scientific research. Scientific research should be the foundation of any publication or recommendation concerning health.

Reliable information can be found in many publications from government agencies, health care foundations, and universities. When we developed the eyefoods plan, we consulted Canada's Food Guide, the Heart and Stroke Foundation's diet and lifestyle recommendations, the Canadian Cancer Society's diet and lifestyle recommendations, and current scientific studies in the field of nutrition and eye health.[84] Furthermore, a registered dietitian reviewed and verified the information in the eyefoods plan.

The eyefoods plan is meant to be included as part of a healthy lifestyle. You will need to consume more food on a weekly basis than what we recommend in the eyefoods plan. For the remainder of your food intake, follow the guidelines set by Canada's Food Guide.

Weekly Targets

Eyefoods weekly targets:
After careful review of scientific studies, we identified which nutrients are most important in the prevention of eye disease. To determine the recommended intake of each of these nutrients for the eyefoods plan, we paid particular attention to the AREDS study and the Dietary Reference Intakes as recommended by Health Canada.[85] We also studied the nutrient values of hundreds of whole foods and considered how a reasonable diet could include these nutrients. The eyefoods plan is not meant to replace an eye vitamin for those people who are at high risk for eye diseases or who already have diagnosed eye

disease. Rather, this plan is a recommended course of action for leading a lifestyle that promotes eye health and overall physical well-being.

Eyefoods target nutrients: Scientific studies show that the following nutrients may help prevent eye disease. The eyefoods plan includes all of these nutrients.

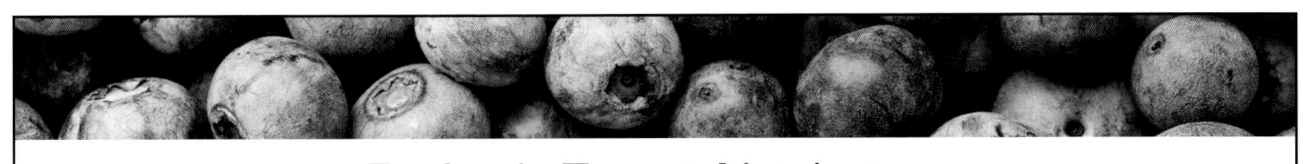

Eyefoods Target Nutrients:

Nutrient	Eyefoods Daily Target	Eyefoods Weekly Target
Lutein and zeaxanthin	10 mg	70 mg
Vitamin C	350 mg	2450 mg
Omega-3 fatty acids from fish (DHA/EPA)	850 mg	5950 mg
Omega-3 fatty acids from plants (ALA)	1600 mg	11 200 mg
Beta-carotene	10 mg	70 mg
Vitamin E	15 mg	105 mg
Zinc	10 mg	70 mg
Fiber	30 grams	210 grams

The Eyefoods Plan   Chapter 5

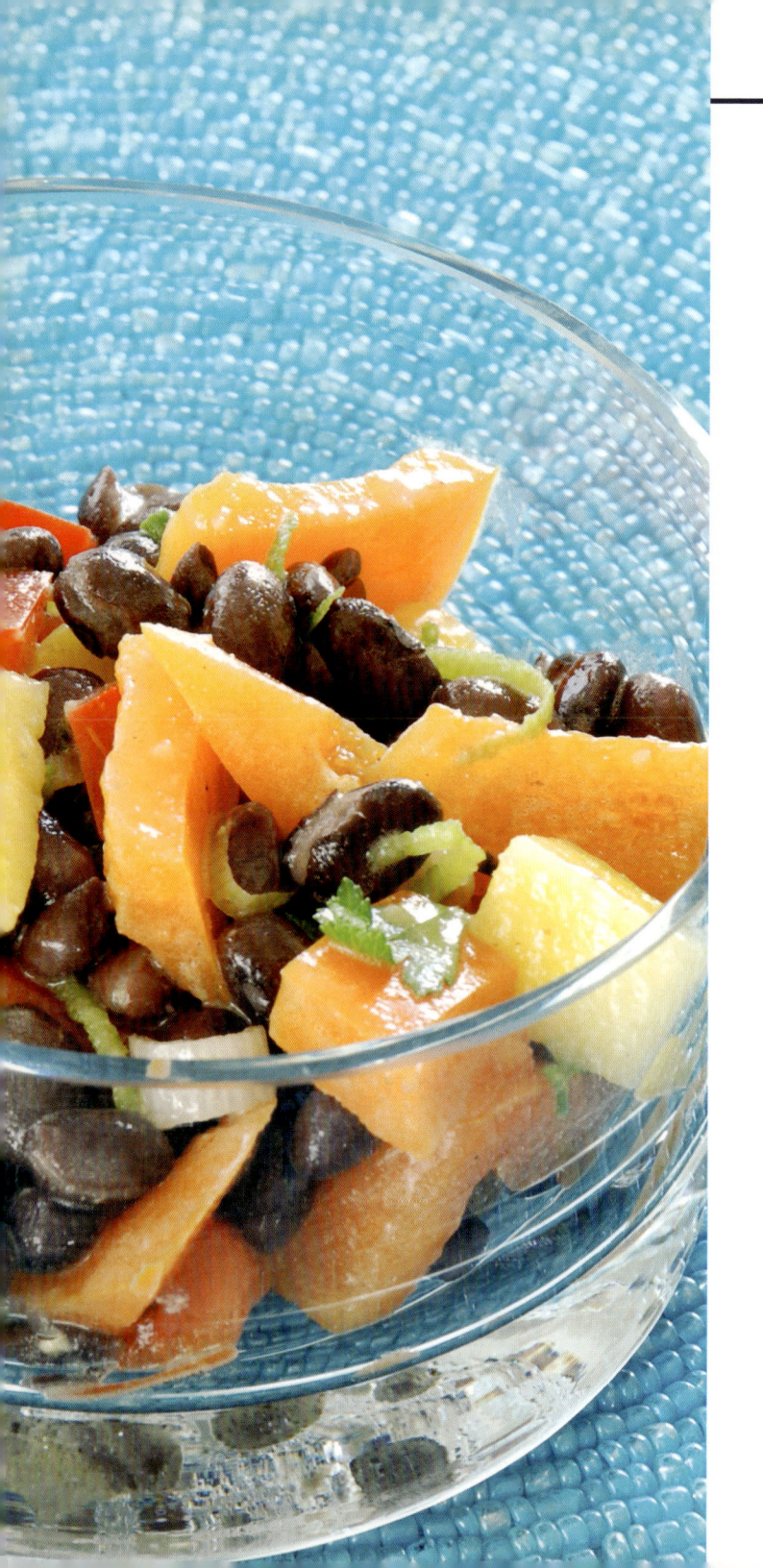

The eyefoods nutrition plan meets all of the weekly targets except zinc. In addition to following the eyefoods nutrition plan, you will need to add whole grains and dairy or dairy-alternative food choices from Canada's Food Guide to your diet. These additional foods will help you to achieve the zinc target.

Serving Sizes

Most nutrition and diet plans offer serving size suggestions that can be confusing. When following a nutrition plan, proper serving sizes are important to ensure that you receive enough of the recommended nutrient in each food. The eyefoods plan recommends serving sizes that allow you to obtain optimal health benefits from each food while maintaining proper portion control.

With our busy lifestyles, we don't usually have time to weigh or measure each food that we eat to determine the proper serving size. The chart below offers simple guidelines that you can use to quickly determine the serving size of certain foods.

Serving Sizes

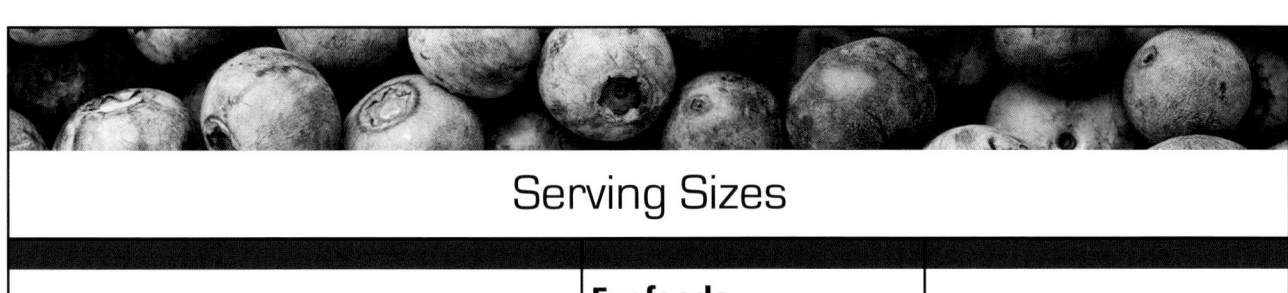

Food	Eyefoods Serving Size	Handy Tips
Raw leafy green vegetables	1 cup	1 large handful
Other vegetables	½ cup	Size of a small lemon
Fruit	1 medium fruit or ½ cup	Size of a small lemon
Fish and lean protein	100 grams	Size of a deck of cards
Nuts	16 grams	1 small handful
Whole grains	½ cup cooked or 1 thin slice of bread	Size of a small lemon
Oil	1 tablespoon	

The Eyefoods Plan   Chapter 5

The Eyefoods Nutrition Plan

Category	Foods	Target
Cooked leafy green vegetables	Kale, spinach, dandelion greens, Swiss chard, other leafy green vegetables	Eat ½ cup twice per week.
Raw leafy green vegetables	Kale, spinach, radicchio, romaine, other dark green lettuce	Eat 7 cups per week. Choose kale and spinach often.
Cold water fish	Wild salmon, sardines, mackerel, tuna, rainbow trout	Eat 2 wild salmon servings per week. Eat 2 servings of other fish per week.
Cooked orange vegetables	Sweet potato, carrots, canned pumpkin, butternut squash	Eat ½ cup three times per week.
Raw carrots	Carrot sticks, shredded carrot, carrot juice	Eat ½ cup three times per week.
Orange peppers	Orange peppers	Eat ½ pepper four times per week.
Green vegetables	Raw broccoli, Brussels sprouts, peas, green beans	Eat ½ cup seven times per week.
Eggs	Eggs high in omega-3 fatty acids.	Eat 2 eggs twice per week. (Total 4 eggs per week)

The Eyefoods Nutrition Plan

Category	Foods	Target
Fruit	Kiwi, cantaloupe, avocado, apricots (dried and fresh), berries, citrus, other fruit	Eat 3 servings per day. (Each serving is ½ cup, or 1 medium fruit, or 4 dried apricots.)
Juice	Orange juice, apple juice, lemon juice	Drink 1 cup juice per day. Add 2 tbsp lemon juice to water or tea per day.
Lean protein	Turkey breast, lean cuts of beef	Eat 400 g turkey breast and 200 g lean beef per week.
Nuts and seeds	Eyefoods nut mix, flax seed, wheat germ	Eat 1 small handful eyefoods nut mix per day, plus 1 tbsp ground flax seed or wheat germ per day.
Whole grains	Oatmeal and bran cereal	Eat ¾ cup five times per week.
Beans and lentils	Black beans, Romano beans, kidney beans, chick peas, white beans, lentils	Eat ½ cup beans or lentils four times per week.
Soy	Edamame	Eat ½ cup twice per week.
Oil	Olive oil, canola oil	2 tbsp olive oil or canola oil per day.

The Eyefoods Plan   Chapter 5

Track It

Food	Eat This Many Servings Weekly
Cooked leafy greens	●●
Raw leafy greens	●●●●●●●
Cold water fish	●●●●
Cooked orange vegetables	●●●
Raw carrots	●●●
Orange peppers	●●●●
Green vegetables	●●●●●●●
Eggs	●●●●
Fruit	●●●●●●● ●●●●●●● ●●●●●●●
Juice	●●●●●●●
Lean protein	●●●●●●
Nuts and seeds	●●●●●●●
Whole grains	●●●●●
Beans and lentils	●●●●
Soy (edamame)	●●
Canola or olive oil	●●●●●● ●●●●●●●

Part 3   The Plan

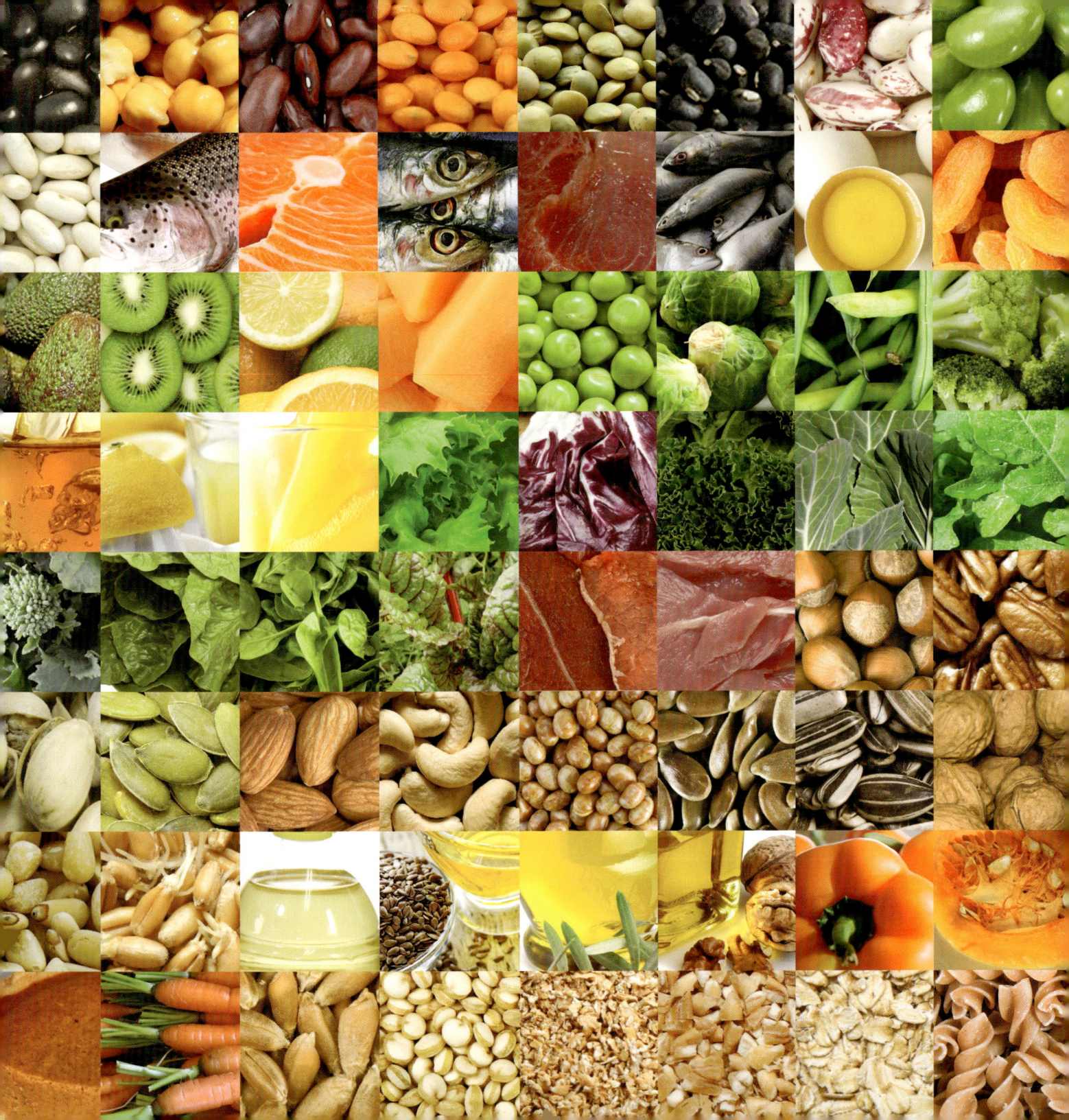

The Eyefoods Lifestyle Plan

Follow the eyefoods nutrition plan.

Wear good-quality sunglasses. See your eye care professional for advice on the best type of sunglasses for you.

Take control of your health. Seek out the services of an eye care professional, a family physician, and any other necessary health care providers. Visit them regularly and have them work as a team for you.

Get moving. Exercise daily. Go for a walk or a bike ride, dance with your family, and learn a new sport or activity. It will bring balance to your life and make you smile more!

Quit smoking. Visit Health Canada's website (http://www.hc-sc.gc.ca/hc-ps/tobac-tabac/quit-cesser/now-maintenant/index-eng.php[86]) or consult your family physician for help.

Take an eye vitamin. If you are at risk for developing eye disease, have eye disease, or cannot reach the eyefoods targets through your diet, take an eye vitamin. Consult your eye care provider regarding the best supplement for you.

Maintain a healthy weight. If you follow the eyefoods lifestyle and nutrition plan, you will be on your way to achieving this goal.

Part 3   The Plan

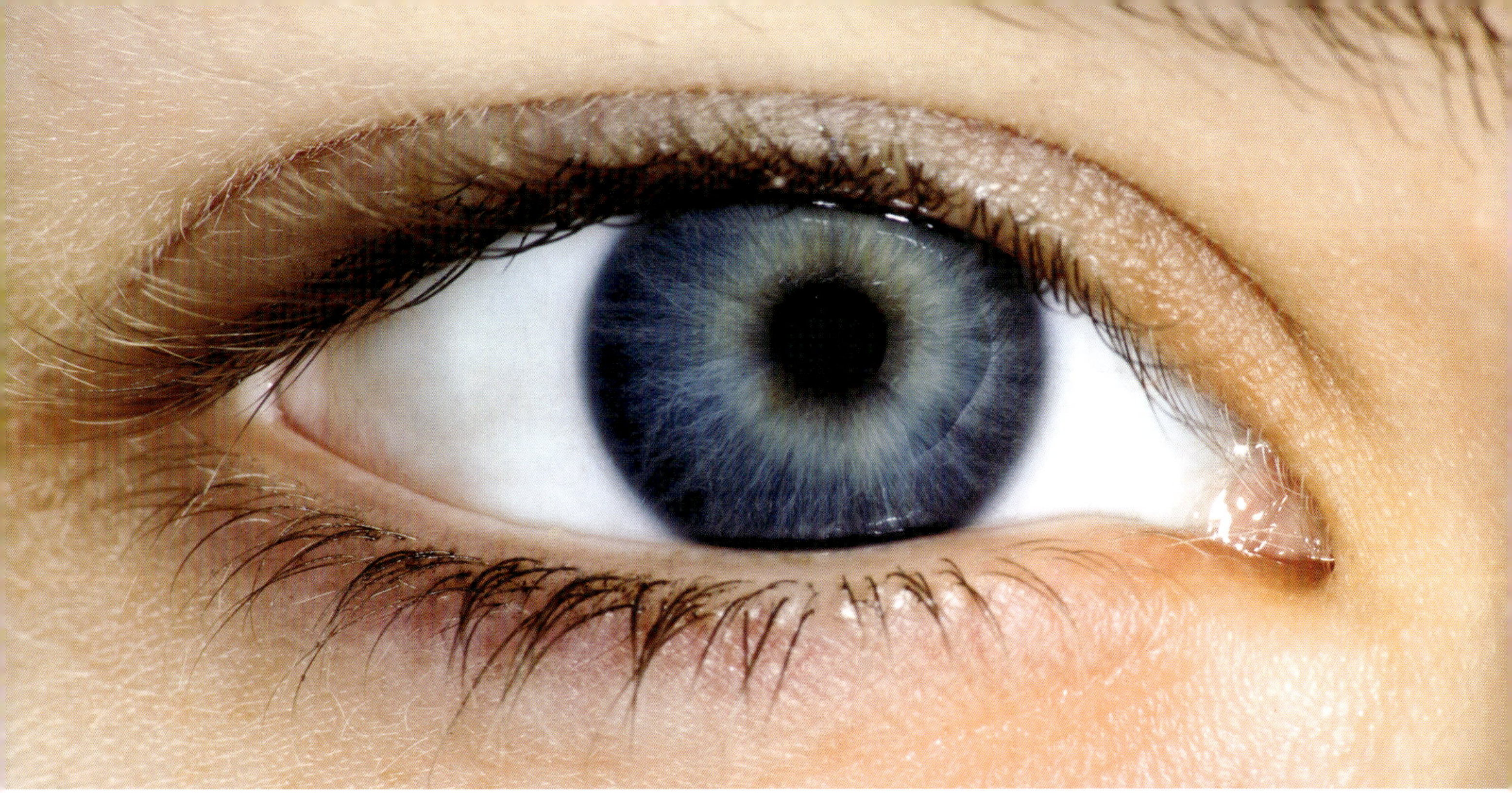

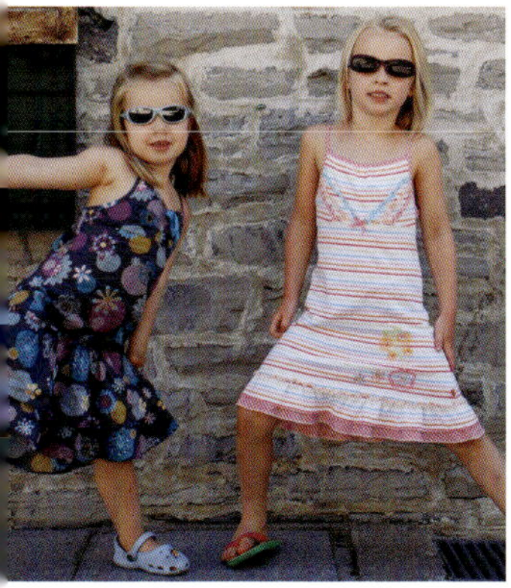

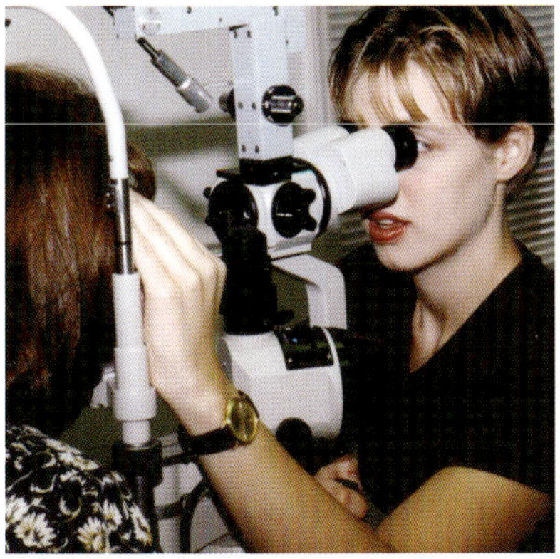

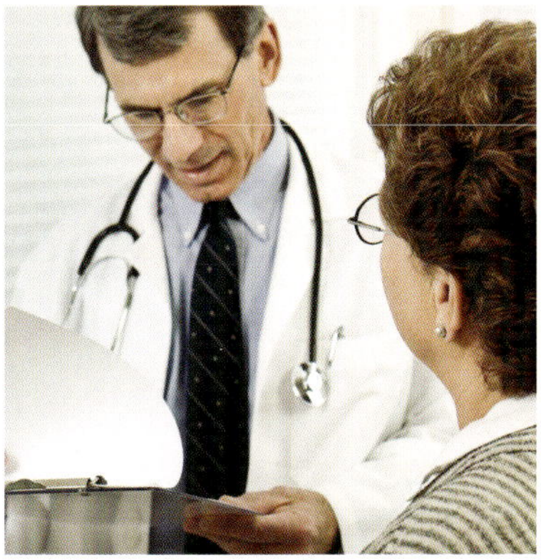

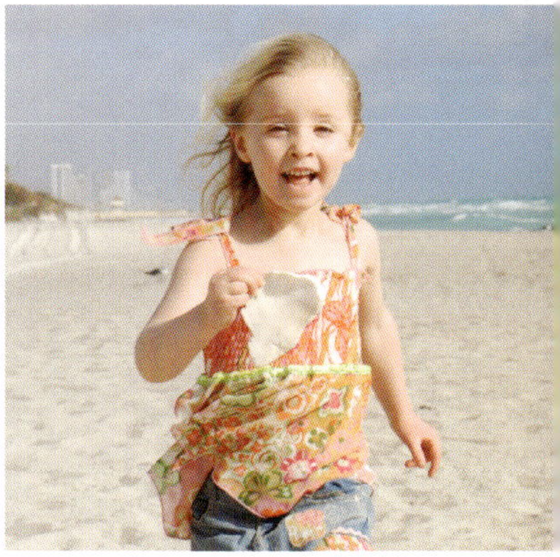

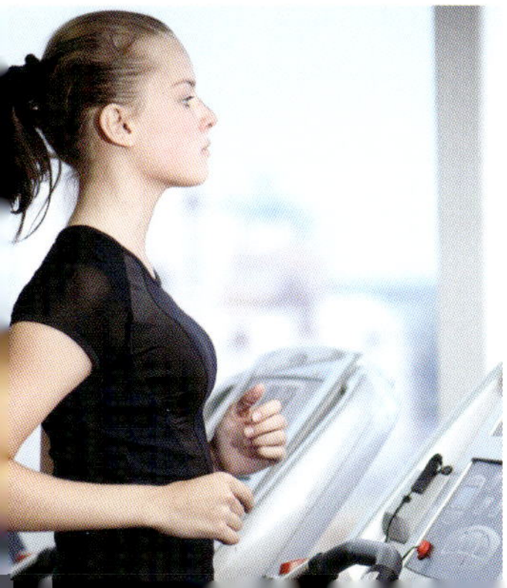

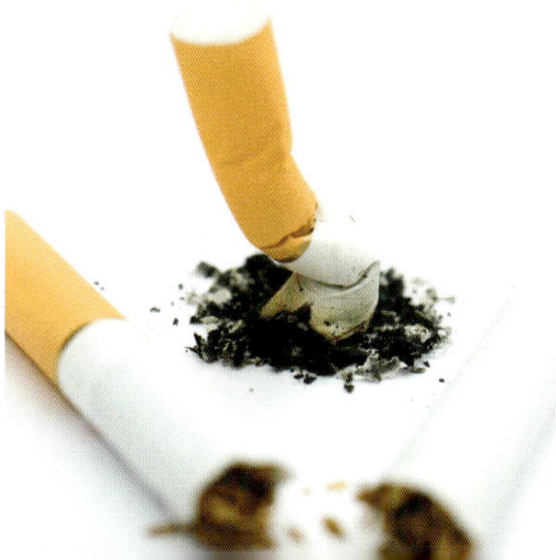

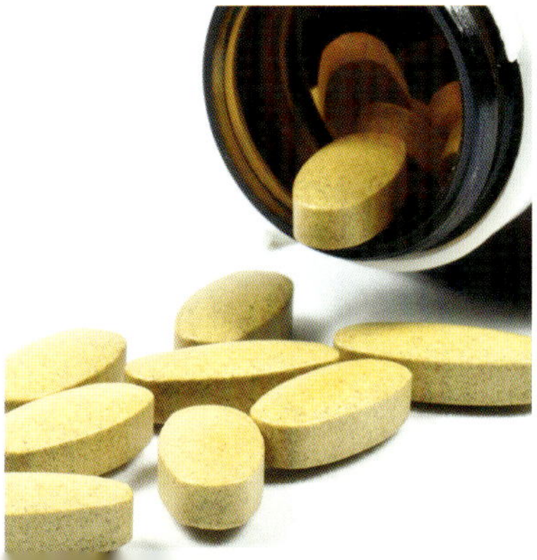

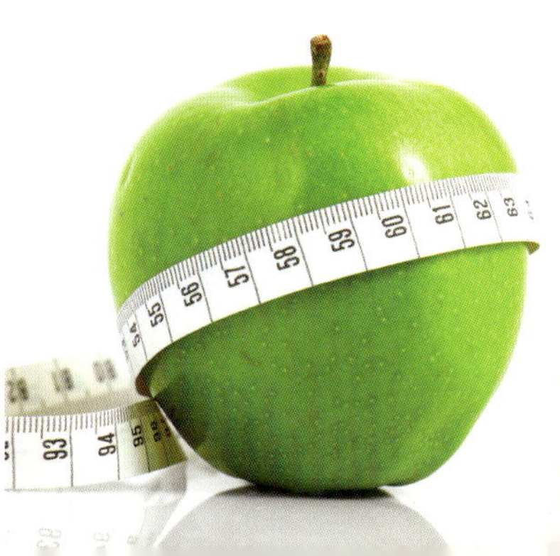

Eyefood for Thought

The eyefoods nutrition plan and the eyefoods lifestyle plan include benefits from food and lifestyle activities that are supported by current scientific studies to promote healthy eyes and reduce the risk of certain eye disease. As is the case with health and medical information, new scientific research is continually emerging regarding other nutrients and lifestyle factors that can help to fight eye disease. In addition to those nutrients that we recommend in the eyefoods plan, other nutrients have shown a relationship with eye disease in early scientific studies.

Emerging Research[87]

An early study on resveratrol, a substance found in red wine and the skin of red grapes, shows a possible improvement in age-related macular degeneration when taken in supplement form. Most of the current studies on resveratrol use animal models or have a small number of human study participants, so larger studies with human subjects are necessary to confirm the benefit of resveratrol on eye health. However, these initial findings are very promising and resveratrol may become a powerful substance in the fight against age-related macular degeneration and, possibly, other eye diseases.

Flavonoids, a class of plant compounds, are known to be beneficial in the prevention of cancer. Emerging research on flavonoids suggests that they may also offer a benefit to people with certain diseases of the retina.

The Future of Eyefoods

We are committed to a lifetime of eyefoods. As new scientific research emerges regarding nutrition, lifestyle, and eye health and disease, we will continue to build upon the eyefoods foundation that we formed in *Eyefoods: A Food Plan for Healthy Eyes*.

Future *Eyefoods* publications will include a more in-depth look at the benefits of these other nutrients as new findings are discovered. We will also provide new and exciting ways to help integrate eyefoods into your life, including fresh recipes and meal plans.

Eyefood for Thought

Acknowledgements

We would like to thank our husbands, parents, and families for their support during the process of making this book. Your encouragement and insight have been invaluable.

Special thanks to our contributors: Liz, Erin, and Rose, who showed great enthusiasm and professionalism while working with us on *Eyefoods: A Food Plan for Healthy Eyes*. Our "baby" would not be the same if we didn't have your help.

Thank you Henri-Louis St-Martin, M.A., Chantal Nanini, Ph. D. and Gaston Bérubé, O.D. for your help, advice and support.

Thank you Dr. Taylor and Dr. Jean for your kind words.

Thank you to our inquisitive patients who have inspired us to research and write about this topic.

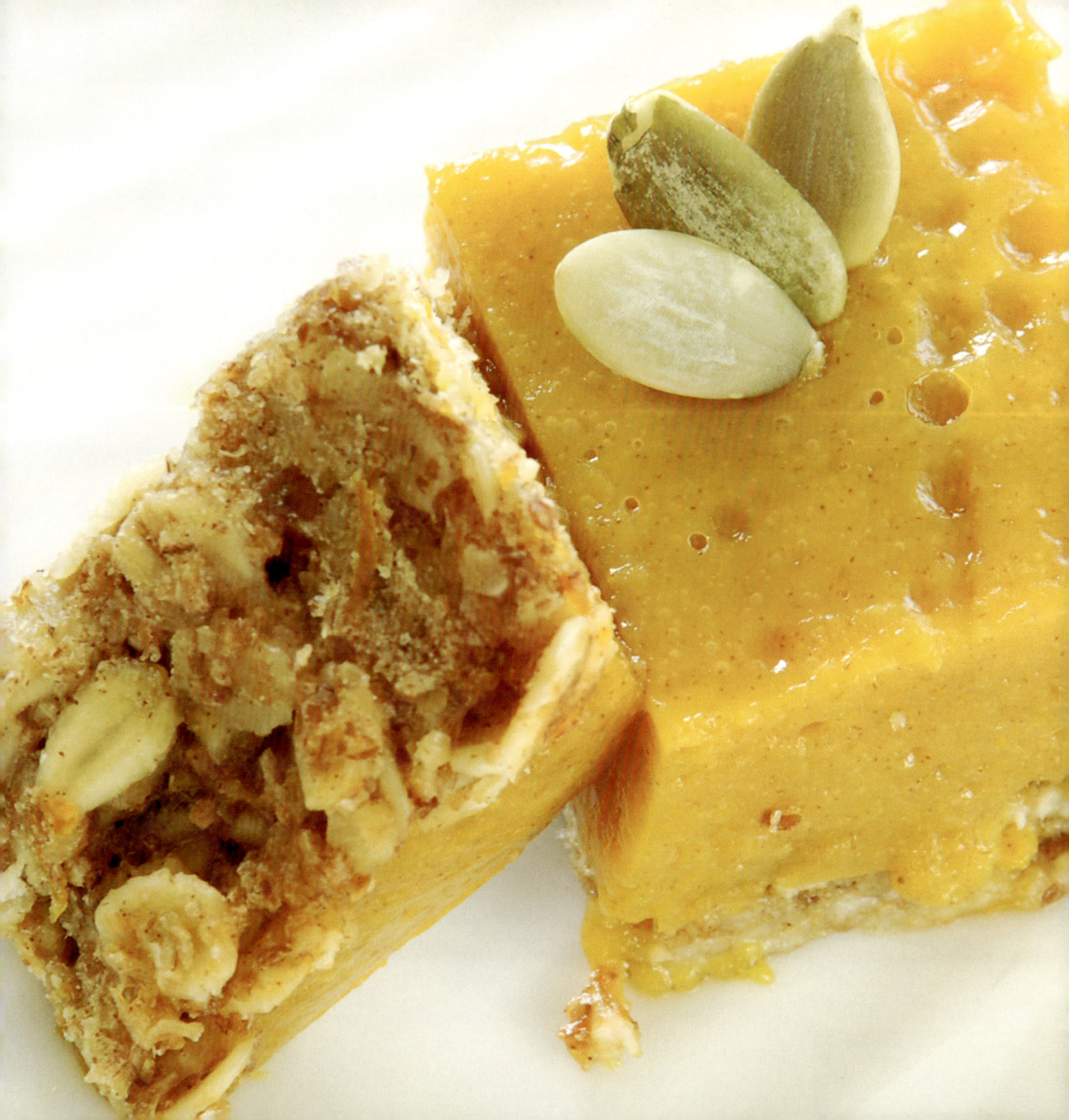

Glossary

Acne rosacea: Facial skin redness caused by hundreds of tiny dilated blood vessels near the surface of the facial skin that become inflamed or dilated.

Adequate intake (AI): The estimated average intake of a nutrient for a healthy population.

Age-related macular degeneration (AMD): A disease of the retina that causes loss of central vision.

Alpha-linolenic acid (ALA): A plant-derived omega-3 fatty acid.

Amsler grid: A vision test used to detect distortion of central vision, indicating possible changes in the macula.

Anterior cortical cataract: A clouding of the front surface of the eye's lens.

Anti-reflective coating: A treatment for optical lenses that removes most glare from glasses and improves visual performance.

Anti-VEGF (vaso endothelial growth factor) injections: An injection of medication into the eye to help stop bleeding or fluid leakage in the retina.

Antioxidant: A class of vitamins and nutrients that helps to prevent oxidation in the body.

AREDS (Age-related eye disease study): A large randomized controlled study on the effects of antioxidants (such as beta-carotene, vitamin C, vitamin E, and zinc) on the prevention of age-related macular degeneration.

AREDS-2 (Age-related eye disease study 2): An ongoing study on the effects of lutein, zeaxanthin, and omega-3 fatty acids on the prevention of age-related macular degeneration.

Artificial teardrops: Lubrication drops used in the treatment of dry eye syndrome or ocular surface disease.

Beta-carotene: An antioxidant of the carotenoid family.

Blepharitis: An ocular condition characterized by chronic inflammation of the eyelid margin.

Blue light: Short-wavelength visible light of blue color, which is close in wavelength to UV light and may cause damage to the eyes.

Body Mass Index (BMI): Ratio of weight to height. BMI = weight (kg)/ height (m)^2.

Bounce-back glare: The reflection of sunlight on the back surface of an optical lens into the eye.

Canada's Food Guide: A document issued by Health Canada containing nutritional recommendations for Canadians.

Canada's Physical Activity Guide: A document issued by Health Canada containing exercise recommendations for Canadians.

Glossary

Canadian Association of Optometrists: A nationwide group representing optometrists across Canada.

Cardiovascular disease: Various medical conditions that affect the heart and blood vessels.

Carotenoid: A naturally occurring pigment that gives fruits and vegetables their color.

Cataract: An ocular condition characterized by a clouding of the lens in the eye.

Cataract surgery: A surgical procedure in which the natural, clouded lens of the eye is removed and replaced by an intraocular lens implant.

Chalazion: A chronic stye in which the previously infected meibomian gland becomes a fibrous dense mass.

Choroid: The tissue behind the retina in the eye. It is the blood supply of the retina.

Dietary reference intakes (DRI): A group of reference values issued by the Institute of Medicine that is useful to determine the adequate nutrient intake for a healthy population.

Direct glare: Glare that originates directly from the sun above and from its reflection below.

Docosahexaenoic acid (DHA): A fish-derived omega-3 fatty acid.

Drusen: Calcifications that form in the retina. An early sign of age-related macular degeneration.

Glossary

Dry age-related macular degeneration (dry AMD): A form of age-related macular degeneration that is characterized by the presence of drusen and pigment changes in the retina.

Dry eye syndrome: A common ocular condition characterized by an imbalance in the tear film.

Eicosapentaenoic acid (EPA): A fish-derived omega-3 fatty acid.

Eyelid hygiene: The practice of using a product to cleanse the eyelids and the base of the eyelashes. Used in the treatment of eyelid disorders.

Fiber: The portion of fruits and vegetables that our body is unable to digest. Adequate fiber intake is essential for a healthy diet.

Glycemic index: A measure of how much an individual food raises the glucose level in the blood compared to a standard food.

Glycemic load: A measure of the glycemic index of a food in relation to its carbohydrate content.

Health Canada: A department of the federal government of Canada that is responsible for helping Canadians maintain and improve their health.

Hyperopia: A condition of the eye where the ocular image is focused behind the eye. Also known as farsightedness.

Inflammation: The body's response to invaders such as bacteria or viruses. It is essential to the healing process.

Glossary

Insoluble fiber: A plant compound that absorbs water through the digestive tract and helps maintain healthy bowels.

Institute of Medicine (IOM): An independent non-profit organization that works outside of government in the United States to provide unbiased and authoritative advice to decision makers and the public.

Intraocular lens implants: Lenses that are implanted in the eye during cataract surgery to replace the natural lens and allow a person to achieve clear vision while minimizing the need for glasses or contact lenses.

Laser photocoagulation: Laser treatment used for the treatment of various eye diseases of the retina, including age-related macular degeneration and retinal holes and tears.

Lid scrubs: Used in the treatment of eyelid disorders to cleanse the eyelid margins with a special product.

Lipofuscin: Fine yellow-brown pigment granules related to aging tissues in the body. It is thought to be a major risk factor in age-related macular degeneration.

Lutein: A pigment that is abundant in the macula of the eye. The human body cannot make lutein.

Meibomianitis: An eyelid disorder that involves inflammation of the oil glands in the eyelids.

Myopia: An ocular condition where light is focused in front of the retina. Also known as nearsightedness.

Glossary

Nuclear sclerosis: A type of cataract that is characterized by a cloudiness of the middle part of the lens.

Ocular surface disease: An ocular condition characterized by an imbalance of the tear film, also called dry eye syndrome.

Omega-3 fatty acids: A family of unsaturated fatty acids that include EPA, DHA, and ALA.

Omega-6 fatty acids: A family of unsaturated fatty acids that are found in vegetable oil, nuts, and seeds, among other foods.

Omega-6 : Omega-3: A measure of the omega-6 fatty acids intake compared to omega-3 fatty acids intake. An ideal omega-6 to omega-3 ratio is 1:1.

Ophthalmologist: A medical doctor who specializes in the diagnosis and treatment of eye conditions and diseases. Many ophthalmologists are also eye surgeons.

Optician: A registered professional who is specially trained to design, fit, and dispense eyeglasses, contact lenses, low vision aids, and prosthetic ocular devices.

Optometrist: A doctor of optometry who specializes in examining, diagnosing, treating, managing, and preventing diseases and disorders of the visual system.

Oxidation: A chemical reaction that changes a stable molecule into a free radical. Free radicals can contribute to the development of chronic disease in the body.

Phaco-emulsification: A technique used in cataract surgery to remove the natural lens or cataract from the eye.

Photochromic lens: An optical lens that darkens when it is activated by ultraviolet light.

Photodynamic therapy with Visudyne® (verteporfin): A treatment option for wet age-related macular degeneration that involves an intravenous injection of a medication followed by treatment with a low-energy laser.

Polarized lenses: Optical lenses that eliminate glare caused by reflections.

Posterior subcapsular cataract: A cloudiness or opacification of the back surface of the lens.

Presbyopia: An ocular condition in which the focusing ability of the eye decreases. It occurs in all people over the age of 40.

Punctal occlusion: A treatment option for dry eye syndrome that involves blocking the tear ducts in the eyelids. This can be done using collagen or silicone punctal plugs or by cauterization.

Punctal plugs: Devices made out of collagen or silicone that are used in the treatment of dry eye syndrome to block the tear ducts.

Recommended dietary allowance (RDA): The average daily intake of a nutrient that is sufficient to meet the dietary requirements of nearly all healthy individuals of a particular life stage or gender group.

Glossary

Reflected glare: Glare that is produced by flat, smooth, and shiny reflective surfaces.

Refractive error: An ocular condition in which light is not focused directly on the retina. It is myopia, hyperopia, astigmatism, prespbyopia, or a combination of these.

Retina: A complex tissue that lines the back surface of the eye. Light focuses on the retina and the retina sends nerve impulses to the brain, allowing it to perceive the image.

Schirmer tear test: A test used to diagnose dry eye syndrome.

Sjogren's syndrome: A condition that is characterized by dry mucous membranes in the body.

Soluble fiber: Plant compounds that are found in legumes, beans, oats, barley, and some fruits and vegetables.

Staphylococcal bacteria: Bacteria that are commonly found on the surface of the eyelids and eyelashes.

Stye: An acute infection of the meibomian glands in the eyelid.

Tear film: The most external surface of the eye. It is made up of three layers: aqueous, mucous, and oil.

Tolerable upper intake level (UL): The highest daily intake of a nutrient that is likely to have no adverse effects for most people.

UV 400: A coating for optical lenses that blocks UV light.

Glossary

Ultraviolet light (UV): Light that is not visible and that ranges in wavelength from 10 nanometers to 400 nanometers.

Ultraviolet light A (UVA): Long-wavelength UV light that ranges in wavelength from 315 nanometers to 400 nanometers.

Ultraviolet light B (UVB): Medium-wavelength UV light that ranges in wavelength from 280 nanometers to 315 nanometers.

Ultraviolet light C (UVC): Short-wavelength light that ranges in wavelength from 100 nanometers to 280 nanometers.

Visible spectrum: Light waves that are visible to the human eye. The wavelengths range from 400 nanometers to 700 nanometers.

Vitamin C: A water-soluble antioxidant that cannot be made nor stored by the human body. Also known as ascorbic acid.

Vitamin D: A fat-soluble vitamin stored by our bodies. It is synthesized in our skin by ultraviolet B rays in sunlight.

Vitamin E: A fat-soluble antioxidant that comes in eight different forms.

Waist circumference: The diameter of a person's waist as measured at the top of the hip bones with a measuring tape that fits comfortably around the waist without depressing the skin.

Wet age-related macular degeneration (wet AMD): The advanced form of age-related macular degeneration that is characterized by fluid or blood in the retina.

World Health Organization (WHO): The directing and coordinating authority for health within the United Nations system.

Zeaxanthin: A pigment that is abundant in the macula of the eye. The human body cannot make zeaxanthin. It is the nutrient accompaniment to lutein.

Zinc: An essential trace mineral that is critical for growth and development and is present in every cell of our bodies.

Notes

Introduction

1. Seddon, *Multivitamin-multimineral supplements and eye disease*, 304S-307S; Miljanovic, *Relation between dietary n-3 and n-6 fatty acids and clinically diagnosed dry eye syndrome in women*, 887-93.

2. Beliveau, *Cooking with foods that fight cancer.*

Chapter 1 – Eye Health and Disease

3. Eye Disease Prevalence Research Group, *Causes and prevalence of visual impairment among adults in the United States*, 477-85; Somani, *Managing patients at risk for age-related macular degeneration: a Canadian strategy*, 14-20.

4. AREDS, *A randomized, placebo-controlled, clinical trial of high-dose supplementation*, 1417-36; AREDS Research Group, *The relationship of dietary carotenoid and vitamin A, E, and C intake with age-related macular degeneration in a case-control study*, 1225-32.

5. Moeller, *Association between intermediate AMD and lutein and zeaxanthin in CAREDS*, 1151-62; de Jong, *Dietary antioxidant intake reduces the risk of AMD*, 45; AREDS Research Group, *The relationship of dietary omega-3 long-chain polyunsaturated fatty acid intake with incident age-related macular degeneration*, 1274-9; Augood, *Oily fish consumption, dietary docosahexaenoic acid and eicosapentaenoic acid intakes*, 398-406; Seddon, *Progression of ARM associated with BMI*, 121, 785-92.

6. Kaushik, *Dietary glycemic index and the risk of age-related macular degeneration*, 1104-10; Seddon, *Obesity linked to increased risk of AMD progression.*

7. Brown, *Anti-VEGF agents in the treatment of neovascular age-related macular degeneration*, 627-37.

8. Klein, *Further observations on the association between smoking and the long-term incidence and progression of age-related macular degeneration*, 115-21.

9. Chiu, *AREDS dietary carbohydrate and glycemic index in relation to cortical and nuclear lens opacities*, 1177-84; Tan, *Carbohydrate nutrition, glycemic index, and the 10-year incidence of cataract*, 1502-8.

10 Tan, *Antioxidant nutrient intake and the long-term incidence of age-related cataract,* 1899-905; Moeller, *Associations between age-related nuclear cataract and lutein and zeaxanthin in the diet and serum in CAREDS,* 354-64; Jacques, *Long-term nutrient intake and early age-related nuclear lens opacities,* 1009-19; Chasan-Taber, *A prospective study of carotenoids and vitamin A intakes and risk of cataract extraction in US women,* 509-16; Townend, *Dietary macronutrients and five-year incident cataract,* 932-39.

11 Pinheiro, *Oral flax seed oil (linum usitatissimum) in the treatment for dry-eye Sjogren's syndrome patients,* 649-55; Miljanovi, *Relation between dietary n-3 and n-6 fatty acids and clinically diagnosed dry eye syndrome in women,* 887-93.

12 Calder, *N-3 Polyunsaturated fatty acids, inflammation, and inflammatory diseases,* S1505-1519.

13 Calder, *N-3 Polyunsaturated fatty acids, inflammation, and inflammatory diseases,* S1505-1519; Beliveau, *Cooking with foods that fight cancer.*

Chapter 2 – Eye Nutrients

14 *Consumer's Guide to DRIs.*

15 Carpentier, *Associations between lutein, zeaxanthin, and age-related macular degeneration,* 313-26; Seddon, *Multivitamin-multimineral supplements and eye disease,* 304S-307S.

16 McDermott, *Antioxidant Nutrients,* 785-99.

17 Nutrient values for orange peppers were obtained through a commissioned study conducted by Maxxam Analytics (Mississauga, ON) for the Guelph Food Technology Centre.

18 Roodenburg, *Amount of fat in the diet affects bioavailability of lutein esters,* 1187–93; Agricultural Research Service, *Nutrient data laboratory.*

19 Richer, *Double-masked, placebo-controlled, randomized trial of lutein and antioxidant supplementation in the intervention of atrophic AMD,* 216-30; Moeller, *Associations between intermediate AMD and lutein and zeaxanthin in CAREDS,* 1151-62; Seddon, *Dietary carotenoids, vitamins A, C and E, and advanced AMD,* 1413-20; Chasan-Taber, *A prospective study of carotenoid and vitamin A intakes and risk of cataract extraction in US women,* 509-16.

20 Van de Leun, *UV Radiation from sunlight,* 237-44; Morganti, *Role of topical and nutritional supplement to modify the oxidative stress,* 331-9; Voutilainen, *Carotenoids and cardiovascular health,* 1265-71; Sato, *Prospective study of carotenoids, tocopherols, and retinoid concentrations and the risk of breast cancer,* 451-7.

Notes

21 Van Leeuwen, *Dietary intake of antioxidants and risk of AMD,* 3101-7; Tan, *Antioxidant nutrient intake and the long-term incidence of age-related cataracts,* 1899-905; Jacques, *Long-term nutrient intake and early age-related nuclear lens opacities,* 1009-19.

22 McDermott. Antioxidant nutrients, 785-99.

23 Ibid.

24 Johnson, *Potential role of dietary n-3 fatty acids in the prevention of dementia and macular degeneration,* 1494S-8S.

25 Chua, *Dietary fatty acids and the five-year incidence of ARM,* 981-6; Cho, *Prospective study of dietary fat and the risk of AMD,* 209-18; San Giovanni, *The relationship of dietary lipid intake and AMD in a case-control study,* 671-9; Townend, *Dietary macronutrient intake and five-year incident cataracts,* 932-9; Miljanovic, *Relation between dietary n-3 and n-6 fatty acids and clinically diagnosed dry eye syndrome in women,* 887-93; Pinheiro, *Oral flax seed oil (linum usitatissimum) in the treatment for dry-eye Sjogren's syndrome patients,* 649-55.

26 American Heart Association, *Fish 101;* Johnson, *Potential role of dietary n-3 fatty acids in the prevention of dementia and macular degeneration,* 1494-8S; Oh, *Practical applications of fish oil (omega-fatty acids) in primary care,* 28-36.

27 Miljanovic, *Relation between dietary n-3 and n-6 fatty acids and clinically diagnosed dry eye syndrome in women,* 887-93.

28 Oh, *Practical applications of fish oil (omega-fatty acids) in primary care,* 28-36.

29 McDermott. Antioxidant nutrients, 785-799.

30 Van Leeuwen, *Dietary intake of antioxidants and risk of AMD,* 3101-7; Christen, *Dietary carotenoids, vitamins C and E, and risk of cataract in women,* 102-9.

31 McDermott. Antioxidant nutrients, 785-99.

32 Miller, *Meta-analysis: High-dosage vitamin E supplementation may increase all-cause mortality.*

33 National Institute of Health, *Health professional's fact sheet.*

34 Tan, *Dietary antioxidants and long-term incidence of ARMD,* 334-41; AREDS, *A randomized, placebo-controlled, clinical trial of high-dose supplementation,* 1417-36.

35 National Institute of Health, *Health professional's fact sheet.*

36 Ibid.

37 McDermott. Antioxidant nutrients, 785-99.

Notes

38 Tan, *Antioxidant nutrient intake and the long-term incidence of age-related cataracts,* 1899-905; AREDS, *A randomized, placebo-controlled, clinical trial of high-dose supplementation,* 1417-36.

39 McDermott. Antioxidant nutrients, 785-99.

40 Ibid.

41 National Institute of Health, *Health Professional's Fact Sheet.*

42 Parekh, *Association between vitamin D and AMD,* 661-9.

43 National Institute of Health, *Dietary Supplement Fact Sheet*.

44 Ibid.

45 American Heart Association. *Whole Grains and Fiber.*

46 Chiu, *Dietary carbohydrate intake and glycemic index in relation to cortical and nuclear lens opacities in AREDS,* 1177-84; Tan, *Carbohydrate nutrition, glycemic index, and the 10-year incidence of cataracts,* 1502-8; Tan, *AMD and mortality from cardiovascular disease or stroke,* 509-12.

47 Jenkins, *Glycemic index: overview of implications in health and disease,* 266S-73S; Foster-Powell, *International tables of glycemic index,* 871S-93S.

48 Jenkins, *Glycemic index: overview of implications in health and disease,* 266S-73S.

49 Tan, *Carbohydrate nutrition, glycemic index, and the 10-year incidence of cataracts,* 1502-8; Chiu, *Dietary carbohydrate and glycemic index in relation to cortical and nuclear lens opacities in AREDS,* 1177-84; Chiu, *Dietary carbohydrate and the progression of AMD,* 1210-18.

50 Jenkins, *Glycemic index: overview of implications in health and disease,* 266S-73S; Willett, *Glycemic index, glycemic load, and risk of type 2 diabetes,* 274-80S.

Chapter 3 – Eyefoods

51 All nutrient information is from USDA Agricultural Research Service, *Nutrient data laboratory*. Canada's Food Guide information is from Health Canada, *Canada's food guide 2007.*

52 Chitchumroonchokchai, *Assessment of lutein bioavailability from meals and a supplement,* 2280-6; *Handbook of clinical nutrition.*

53 Warren Grant Magnuson Clinical Center, *Important drug and food information.*

54 Roodenburg, *Amount of fat in the diet affects bioavailability of lutein esters,* 1187–93.

55 San Giovanni, *The relationship of dietary lipid intake and AMD in a case-control study,* 671-679; Townend, *Dietary macronutrient intake*

Notes

and 5-year incident cataracts, 932-39; Miljanovic, *Relation between dietary n-3 and n-6 fatty acids and clinically diagnosed dry eye syndrome in women*, 887-93; Oh, *Practical applications of fish oil (omega-3 fatty acids) in primary care*, 28-36.

56 Health Canada, *Health Canada advises specific groups to limit their consumption of canned albacore tuna.*

57 Health Canada, *Prenatal nutrition guidelines for health professionals.*

58 McDermott, *Antioxidant nutrients*, 785-99.

59 Maxxam Analytics. Nutrient values for orange peppers.

60 Chung, *Lutein bioavailablity is higher from lutein-enriched eggs than from supplements and spinach in men*, 1887-93.

61 Hu, *A prospective study of egg consumption and risk of cardiovascular disease in men and women*, 1387-94; Djousse, *Egg consumption in relation to cardiovascular disease and mortality*, 964-9; Qureshi, *Regular egg consumption does not increase the risk of stroke and cardiovascular diseases*, CR1-8.

62 American Heart Association, *How do I follow a healthy diet?*

63 Seddon, *Progression of age-related macular degeneration*, 1728-37

64 Chiu, *Dietary carbohydrate and the progression of age-related macular degeneration*, 1210-18; Chiu, *Dietary carbohydrate intake and glycemic index in relation to cortical and nuclear lens opacities in AREDS*, 1177-84; Tan, *Carbohydrate nutrition, glycemic index, and the 10-year incidence of cataracts*, 1502-8.

65 Tan, *Age-related macular degeneration and mortality from cardiovascular disease or stroke*, 509-12.

66 American Heart Association, *Whole grains and fiber.*

67 Pinheiro, *Oral flax seed oil (Linum usitatissimum) in the treatment for dry-eye Sjogren's syndrome patients.* 649-55.

Chapter 4 – Lifestyle and Eye Health

68 Health Canada, *It's your health: ultraviolet radiation from the sun.*

69 Drobek-Slowik, *The potential role of oxidative stress in the pathogenesis of the age-related macular degeneration (AMD)*, 28-37.

70 Fletcher, *Sunlight exposure, antioxidants, and AMD*, 1396-1403.

71 Ibid.

72 Ibid.

Notes

73 Klein, *Further observations on the association between smoking and the long-term incidence and progression of AMD,* 115-21.

74 Ibid.

75 McDermott, *Antioxidant nutrients,* 785-99.

76 Health Canada, *Quit smoking.*

77 Health Canada, *It's your health: obesity.*

78 Health Canada, *Food and nutrition: body mass index (BMI) nomogram.*

79 Ibid.

80 Seddon, *Progression of ARM associated with BMI, waist circumference and waist, hip ratio,* 785-92.

81 Ibid.

82 Public Health Agency of Canada, *Canada's physical activity guide to healthy active living.*

83 Wong, *AMD and risk for stroke,* 98-106; Tan, *AMD and mortality from cardiovascular disease or stroke,* 509-12.

Chapter 5 - The Eyefoods Plan

84 American Heart Association, Nutrition center; Health Canada. Canada's food guide; Canadian Cancer Society, Nutrition and fitness.

85 Health Canada, A consumer's guide to DRIs.

86 Health Canada, Quit smoking.

87 Richer, *Molecular medicine in ophthalmic care,* 695-701; King, *Resveratrol reduces oxidation and proliferation of human retinal pigment epithelial cells via extracellular signal-regulated kinase inhibition,* 143-49; Kubota, *Resveratrol prevents light-Induced retinal degeneration via suppressing activator protein-1 activation;* Hanneken, *Flavonoids protect human retinal pigment epithelial cells from oxidative-stress–induced death,* 3164-77.

Notes

References

Age-Related Eye Disease Study Research Group (AREDS). 2001. A randomized, placebo-controlled, clinical trial of high-dose supplementation with vitamins C and E, beta carotene, and zinc for age-related macular degeneration and vision loss. *Arch ophthalmol* 119: 1417-36.

———. The relationship of dietary carotenoid and vitamin A, E, and C intake with age-related macular degeneration in a case-control study: AREDS Report No. 22. *Arch ophthalmol*. 2007 Sep; 125(9): 1225-32.

———. 2008. The relationship of dietary omega-3 long-chain polyunsaturated fatty acid intake with incident age-related macular degeneration: AREDS report no. 23. *Arch ophthalmol* 126: 1274-9.

Age-Related Eye Disease Study 2. The lutein/zeaxanthin and omega-3 supplementation trial. http://www.areds2.org/.

Agricultural Research Service. Nutrient Data Laboratory. http://www.nal.usda.gov/fnic/foodcomp/search/.

American Heart Association. Fish 101. http://www.americanheart.org/presenter.jhtml?identifier=3071550.

———. How do I follow a healthy diet? http://www.americanheart.org/downloadable/heart/1196282749644FollowHealthyDiet.pdf.

———. Nutrition center. http://www.heart.org/HEARTORG/GettingHealthy/NutritionCenter/Nutrition-Center_UCM_001188_SubHomePage.jsp.

———. Whole Grains and Fiber.
http://www.americanheart.org/presenter.jhtml?identifier=4574.

Augood, C., U. Chakravarthy, I. Young, J. Vioque, P. de Jong, G. Bentham, M. Rahu, J. Seland, G. Soubrane, L. Tomazzoli, F. Topouzis, J. Vingerling, and A. Fletcher. 2008. Oily fish consumption, dietary docosahexaenoic acid and eicosapentaenoic acid intakes, and associations with neovascular age-related macular degeneration. *Am J Clin Nutr* Aug, 88 (2): 398-406.

Beliveu, R., and D. Gingras. 2006. *Cooking with foods that fight cancer*. Toronto, Ontario: McClelland & Stewart.

Brown, D., and C. Regillo. 2007. Anti-VEGF agents in the treatment of neovascular age-related macular degeneration: Applying clinical trial results to the treatment of everyday patients. *Am J Ophthalmol* Oct, 144 (4): 627-37.

Cackett, P. and T. Wong. 2008. Age-related macular degeneration and mortality from cardiovascular disease or stroke. *Br J Ophthalmol* Nov, 92 (11): 1564.

Calder, P. 2006. N-3 Polyunsaturated fatty acids, inflammation, and inflammatory diseases. *Am J Clin Nutr* 83 (6): S1505-19.

Canadian Cancer Society. Nutrition and fitness.
http://www.cancer.ca/Ontario/Prevention/Eat%20well.aspx?sc_lang=en

Carpentier, S., M. Knaus, and M. Suh. 2009. Associations between lutein, zeaxanthin, and age-related macular degeneration: An overview. *Crit Rev Food Sci Nutr* Apr, 49 (4): 313-26.

Chasan-Taber, L. and W. Willett, J. Seddon, M. Stampfer, B. Rosner, G. Colditz, F. Speizer, and S. Hankinson. 1999. A prospective study of carotenoid and vitamin A intakes and risk of cataract extraction in US women. *Am J Clin Nutr* 70 (4): 509-16.

Chitchumroonchokchai, C., S. Schwartz, and M. Failla. 2004. Assessment of lutein bioavailability from meals and a supplement using simulated digestion and caco-2 human intestinal cells. *J. Nutr* 134: 2280-6.

Chiu, C., R. Milton, R. Klein, G. Gensler, and A. Taylor. 2007. Dietary carbohydrate and the progression of age-related macular degeneration: a prospective study from the age-related eye disease study. *Am J Clin Nutr* 86: 1210-18.

Chiu, C., R. Milton, G. Gensler, and A. Taylor. 2006. Dietary carbohydrate intake and glycemic index in relation to cortical and nuclear lens opacities in the age-related eye disease study. *Am J Clin Nutr* May, 83: 1177-84.

Cho, E, S. Hung, W. Willett, D. Spiegelman, E. Rimm, J. Seddon, G. Colditz, and S. Hankinson. 2001. Prospective study of dietary fat and the risk of AMD. *Am J Clin Nutr* Feb, 73 (2): 209-18.

Christen, W., S. Liu, R. Glynn, J. Gaziano, and J. Buring. 2008. Dietary carotenoids, vitamins C and E, and risk of cataract in women: a prospective study. *Arch ophthalmol* 126 (1): 102-9.

Chua, B., V. Flood, E. Rochtchina, J. Wang, W. Smith, and P. Mitchell. 2006. Dietary fatty acids and the five-year incidence of ARM. *Arch Ophthalmol* 124: 981-6.

Chung, H., H. Rasmussen, and E. Johnson. 2004. Lutein bioavailablity is higher from lutein-enriched eggs than from supplements and spinach in men. *J Nutr* 134 (8) : 1887-93.

De Jong, P., R. van Leeuwen, C. Klaver, J. Vingerling, J. Witteman, S. Boekhoorn, and A. Hofman. 2004. Dietary antioxidant intake reduces the risk of AMD, The Rotterdam Study. *Invest Ophthalmol Vis Sci* 45: E-Abstract 2243.

Drobek-Slowik, M., Karczewicz, D., and Safranow, K. 2007. The potential role of oxidative stress in the pathogenesis of the age-related macular degeneration (AMD). *Postepy Hig Med Dosw* 61:28-37 (ISSN: 1732-2693).

Djousse, L. and J. Gaziano. 2008. Egg consumption in relation to cardiovascular disease and mortality: the physicians' health study. *Am J Clin Nutr* Apr, 87(4): 964-9.

Eye Disease Prevalence Research Group. 2004. Causes and prevalence of visual impairment among adults in the United States. *Arch ophthalmol*. 122: 477-85.

Flax Council of Canada 2003. Flax: A Health and Nutrition Primer. www.flaxcouncil.ca

Fletcher, A., G. Bentham, M. Agnew, I. Young, C. Augood, U. Chakravarthy, P. de Jong, M. Rahu, J. Seland, G. Soubrane, L. Tomazzoli, F. Topouzis, J. Vingerling, and J. Vioque. 2008. Sunlight exposure, antioxidants, and age-related macular degeneration. *Arch ophthalmol* 126 (10): 1396-1403.

Foster-Powell, K. and J. Miller. 1995. International tables of glycemic index. *Am J Clin Nutr* 62: 871S-93S.

Hanneken, A., F. Lin, J. Johnson, and P. Maher. 2006. Flavonoids protect human retinal pigment epithelial cells from oxidative-stress–induced death. *Investigative Opth & Vis Sci* 47: 3164-77.

Health Canada. A consumer's guide to DRIs (Dietary Reference Intakes). http://www.hc-sc.gc.ca/fn-an/nutrition/reference/cons_info-guide_cons-eng.php

———. Canada's Food Guide. 2007. http://www.hc-sc.gc.ca/fn-an/food-guide-aliment/index-eng.php.

———. 2003. Food and nutrition: Body mass index (BMI) nomogram, Sept 19. http://www.hc-sc.gc.ca/fn-an/nutrition/weights-poids/guide-ld-adult/bmi_chart_java-graph_imc_java-eng.php.

———. 2007. Health Canada advises specific groups to limit their consumption of canned albacore tuna, March 28. http://www.hc-sc.gc.ca/ahc-asc/media/advisories-avis/_2007/2007_14-eng.php.

———. 2009. Health concerns: Quit smoking, Jan 12. http://www.hc-sc.gc.ca/hc-ps/tobac-tabac/quit-cesser/index-eng.php.

———.2006. It's your health: Obesity, October. http://www.hc-sc.gc.ca/hl-vs/alt_formats/pacrb-dgapcr/pdf/iyh-vsv/life-vie/obes-eng.pdf.

———. 2006. It's your health: Ultraviolet radiation from the sun, August. http://www.hc-sc.gc.ca/hl-vs/iyh-vsv/environ/ultraviolet-eng.php#he.

References

———. 2009. Prenatal nutrition guidelines for health professionals: Fish and omega-3 fatty acids. http://www.hc-sc.gc.ca/fin-an/pubs/nutrition/omega3-eng.php.

Hu, F., M. Stampfer, E. Rimm, J. Manson, A. Ascherio, G. Colditz, B. Rosner, D. Spiegelman, F. Speizer, F. Sacks, C. Hennekens, W. Willett. 1999. A prospective study of egg consumption and risk of cardiovascular disease in men and women. *JAMA* 281 (15): 1387-94.

Jacques, P., L. Chylack Jr., S. Hankinson, P. Khu, G. Rogers, J. Friend, W. Tung, J. Wolfe, N. Padhye, W. Willett, A. Taylor. 2001. Long-term nutrient intake and early age-related nuclear lens opacities. *Arch ophthalmol.* 119 (7): 1009-19.

Jenkins, D., C. Kendall, L. Augustin, S. Franceschi, M. Hamidi, A. Marchie, A. Jenkins, and M. Axelsen. 2002. Glycemic index: overview of implications in health and disease. *Am J Clin Nutr* 76 (suppl): 266S-73S.

Johnson, E. and E. Schaefer. 2006. Potential role of dietary n-3 fatty acids in the prevention of dementia and macular degeneration. *Am J Clin Nutr* 83 (suppl): 1494S-8S.

Kaushik, S., J. Wang, V. Flood, J. Sue, L. Tan, A. Barclay, T. Wong, J. Brand-Miller, and P. Mitchell. 2008. Dietary glycemic index and the risk of age-related macular degeneration. *Am J Clin Nutr* Oct, 88 (4): 1104-10.

King, R., K. Kent, and J. Bomser. 2005. Resveratrol reduces oxidation and proliferation of human retinal pigment epithelial cells via extracellular signal-regulated kinase inhibition. *Chem Biol Interact* Jan 15, 151(2): 143-9.

Klein, R., M. Knudtson, K. Cruickshanks, and B. Klein. 2008. Further observations on the association between smoking and the long-term incidence and progression of age-related macular degeneration: The beaver dam eye study. *Arch ophthalmol* 126 (1): 115-21.

Kubota, S., T. Kurihara, M. Ebinuma, M. Kubota, K. Yuki, M. Sasaki, K. Noda, Y. Ozawa, Y. Oike, S. Ishida, S., and K. Tsubota. 2010. Resveratrol prevents light-induced retinal degeneration via suppressing activator protein-1 activation. *Am J Pathol*, Aug 13. (E-pub ahead of print).

Maxxam Analytics (Mississauga, ON) for the Guelph Food Technology Centre. Commissioned study on nutrient properties of orange peppers. August, 2010.

McDermott, J. 2000. Antioxidant nutrients: Current dietary recommendations and research update. *J Am Pharm Assoc.* 40 (6): 785-99.

Miljanovic, B., K. Trivedi, M. Dana, J. Gilbard, J. Buring, and D. Schaumberg. 2005. Relation between dietary n-3 and n-6 fatty acids and clinically diagnosed dry eye syndrome in women. *Am J Clin Nutr* 82 (4): 887-93.

Miller, E., R. Pastor-Barriuso, D. Dalal, et al. 2004. Meta-analysis: High-dosage vitamin E supplementation may increase all-cause mortality. *Ann Intern Med*; published online before print Nov 10.

Moeller, S., R. Voland, L.Tinker, B. Blodi, M. Klein, K. Gehrs, E. Johnson, D. Snodderly, R. Wallace, R. Chappell, N. Parekh, C. Ritenbaugh, and J. Mares; for the CAREDS Study Group. 2008. Associations between age-related nuclear cataract and lutein and zeaxanthin in the diet and serum in the (CAREDS). *Arch ophthalmol* 126(3): 354-64.

Moeller S., N. Parekh, L. Tinker, C. Ritenbaugh, B. Blodi, R. Wallace, and J. Mares. 2006. Association between intermediate AMD and lutein and zeaxanthin in CAREDS. *Arch ophthalmol* 124: 1151-62.

Morganti, P., C. Bruno, et al. 2002. Role of topical and nutritional supplement to modify the oxidative stress. *Intl J Cosmetic Sci* 24: 331-9.

National Institute of Health. June 2009. Office of dietary supplements: Health professional's fact sheet. http://dietary-Supplements.info.nih.gov/FactSheets/Zinc.asp.

National Institute of Health. Jan 2011. Office of Dietary Supplements: Dietary Supplement Fact Sheet. http://ods.od.nih.gov.factsheets/vitamind/.

References

Oh, R. 2005. Practical applications of fish oil (omega-fatty acids) in primary care. *J Am Board Fam Med* 18 (1): 28-36.

Parekh, N., R. Chappell, A. Millen, D. Albert, J. Mares. 2007. Association between vitamin D and age-related macular degeneration in the third national health and nutrition examination survey, 1988 through 1994. *Arch ophthalmol* 125: 661-9.

Pinheiro Jr, M. dos Santos, P, et al. 2007. Oral flax seed oil (linum usitatissimum) in the treatment for dry-eye Sjogren's syndrome patients. *Arq Bras Oftalmol* 70: 649-55.

Public Health Agency of Canada. Canada's physical activity guide to healthy active living. http://www.phac-aspc.gc.ca/hp-ps/hl-mvs/pa-ap/index-eng.php (January 20, 2011)

Qureshi, A., M. Suri, S. Ahmed, A. Nasar, A. Divani, and J. Kirmani. 2007. Regular egg consumption does not increase the risk of stroke and cardiovascular diseases. *Med Sci Monit* 13 (1): CR1-8.

Richer, S., W. Stiles, L. Statkute, J. Pulido, J. Frankowski, D. Rudy, K. Pei, M. Tsipursky, and J. Nyland. 2004. Double-masked, placebo-controlled, randomized trial of lutein and antioxidant supplementation in the intervention of atrophic age-related macular degeneration: the Veterans LAST study. *Optometry* Apr, 75(4): 216-30.

Richer, S., W. Stiles, C. Thomas. 2009. Molecular medicine in ophthalmic care. *Optometry* Dec, 80 (12): 695-701.

Roodenburg, A., R. Leenen, K. van het Hof, J.Weststrate, and L. Tijburg. 2000. Amount of fat in the diet affects bioavailability of lutein esters but not of alpha-carotene, beta-carotene, and vitamin E in humans. *Am J Clin Nutr*, 71: 1187–93.

San Giovanni, J., E. Chew, T. Clemons, M. Davis, F. Ferris, G. Gensler, N. Kurinij, A. Lindblad, R. Milton, J. Seddon, and R. Sperduto. 2007. The relationship of dietary lipid intake and age-related macular degeneration in a case-control study. AREDS report No. 20. *Arch Ophthalmol* 125 (5): 671-9.

Sato, N., K. Helzlsouer, et al. 2002. Prospective study of carotenoids, tocopherols, and retinoid concentrations and the risk of breast cancer. *Cancer epidermiol biomarkers Prev* 11: 451-7.

Seddon, J., U. Ajani, R. Sperduto, R. Hiller, N. Blair, T. Burton, M. Farber, E. Gragoudas, J. Haller, D. Miller, L. Yannuzzi, W. Willett. 1994. Dietary carotenoids, vitamins A, C and E, and advanced age-related macular degeneration. *JAMA* 272(18): 1413-20.

Seddon, J. 2007. Multivitamin-multimineral supplements and eye disease: Age-related macular degeneration and cataract. *Am J Clin Nutr.* Jan, 85 (1): 304S-307S.

Seddon, J. 2003. Obesity linked to increased risk of AMD progression. *Ocul-Surg-News* 20, Abstract.

Seddon, J., J. Cote, N. Davis, and B. Rosner. 2003. Progression of ARM associated with BMI, waist circumference and waist, hip ratio. *Arch ophthalmol* 121: 785-92.

Seddon, J., J. Cote, and B. Rosner. 2003. Progression of age-related macular degeneration association with dietary fat, transunsaturated fat, nuts and fish intake. *Arch ophthalmol* Dec, 121 (12): 1728-37.

Shweta, K., J. Wang, V. Flood, J. Sue, L. Tan, A. Barclay, T. Wong, J. Brand-Miller, and P. Mitchell. 2008. Dietary glycemic index and the risk of age-related macular degeneration. *Am. J. Clin. Nutr.,* Oct., 88 (4): 1104-1110.

Somani, S., A. Hoskin-Mott, A. Mishra, A. Bois, B. Book, M. Chute, R. Gaucher, and B. Winter. 2009. Managing patients at risk for age-related macular degeneration: A Canadian strategy. *Can J Optom* Mar, 71 (2):14-20.

Tan, A., P. Mitchell, V. Flood, G. Burlutsky, E. Rochtchina, R. Cumming, and J. Wang. 2008. Antioxidant nutrient intake and the long-term incidence of age-related cataract: The blue mountains eye study. *Am J Clin Nutr* Jun, 87 (6): 1899-905.

Tan, J., J. Wang, G. Liew, E. Rochtchina, and P. Mitchell. 2008. Age-related macular degeneration and mortality from cardiovascular disease or stroke. *Br J Ophthalmol*, Nov; 92 (1): 509-12.

Tan, J., J. Wang, V. Flood, S. Kaushik, A. Barclay, J. Brand-Miller, and P. Mitchell. 2007. Carbohydrate nutrition, glycemic index, and the 10-year incidence of cataract. *Am J Clin Nutr* 86 (5): 1502-8.

Tan, J., J. Wang, V. Flood, E. Rochtchina, W. Smith, and P. Mitchell. 2008. Dietary antioxidants and long-term incidence of ARMD: The blue mountain eye study. *Ophthalmology* 115: 334-41.

Townend, B., M. Townend, V. Flood, G. Burlutsky, E. Rochtchina, J. Wang, and P. Mitchell. 2007. Dietary macronutrient intake and 5-year incident cataract: The blue mountains eye study. *Am J Ophthalmol* Jun, 143 (6): 932-9.

USDA Agricultural Research Service. Nutrient data laboratory. http://www.nal.usda.gov/fnic/foodcomp/search/.

Van de Leun, J. 1996. UV radiation from sunlight: summary, conclusions, and recommendations. *J Photochem & Photobiol Biol.* 35: 237-44.

Van Leeuwen, R., S. Boekhoorn, J. Vingerling, J. Witteman, C. Klaver, A. Hofman, and P. de Jong. 2005. Dietary intake of antioxidants and risk of age-related macular degeneration. *JAMA* 294 (24): 3101-7.

Voutilainen S. T. Nurmi, J. Mursu, and T. Rissanen. 2006. Carotenoids and cardiovascular health. *Am J Clin Nutr* Jun 83 (6): 1265-71.

Warren Grant Magnuson Clinical Center. National Institutes of Health Drug-Nutrient Interaction Task Force. Important drug and food information. http://dietary-supplements.info.nih.gov/factsheets/cc/coumadin1.pdf

Willett, W., J. Manson, and S. Liu. 2002. Glycemic index, glycemic load, and risk of type 2 diabetes. *Am J Clin Nutr;* 76 (suppl): 274-80S.

Wong, T., R. Klein, C. Sun, P. Mitchell, D. Couper, H. Lai, L. Hubbard, and A. Sharrett, for the Atherosclerosis Risk in Communities Study. 2006. Age-related macular degeneration and risk for stroke. *Ann Intern Med,* Jul 18, 145 (2):98-106.

Index

age-related macular degeneration (AMD)
    causes, 29, 53, 63
    definition, 29, 34
    diagnosis, 31, 33
    control & prevention with diet, 31, 32, 34, 50, 54, 60, 64, 139
    risk factors, 31, 34, 113–115, 120, 122–123
    symptoms, 31, 34
    treatment, 33–34
    types
        dry and wet AMD, 29, 33, 34
Anti-VEGF medication (vaso-endophelial growth factor), 33
American Heart Association, 57
Amsler grid
    in diagnosis of AMD, 31, 33
antioxidants, 21, 31, 33-34, 49, 55, 59, 61, 79, 88
    definition, 54
    and eye disease, 54, 114
    and general health, 53
Age-related eye disease study (AREDS), 31-34, 128
Age-related eye disease study follow up (AREDS-2), 32, 54, 120
Asian cuisine, 75, 104

beans and lentils, 60, 62, 64, 72, 104–105, 133–134
    chick peas, 104–105, 133
    black beans, 104–105, 133
    lentils, 64, 104–105, 133–134
    kidney beans, 104–105, 133
    romano beans, 104–105
    soybeans (edamame), 95, 104–105, 133–134
    white beans, 104–105, 133
beef, 85, 92–93, 133
beta-carotene, 21, 32, 52–53, 70, 79, 80, 82, 84, 89
    definition, 61
    and eye health, 61
    and general health, 61, 120
    recommended intake, 61, 129
blepharitis & meibomianitis, *see under eyelid disorders*
blindness, 29, 34
blood thinners, 72

blue light
    effect on eye-health, 31, 37, 54, 113–116, 119
body mass index (BMI), 121–122

Canada's Food Guide recommendations, 76, 80, 85–86, 89, 93, 97, 100–101, 110, 128, 130
Canadian Cancer Society, 128
cancer, 21, 45, 53, 55–56, 59, 61–62, 64, 69–70, 74, 79, 114, 116, 120, 128, 139
cardiovascular disease, 31, 53, 64, 69–70, 74, 95, 100–101, 122–123
carotenoids, 21, 32, 35, 36, 38, 53, 54
cataracts, 21
    definition, 35, 38
    diagnosis, 36
    control & prevention with diet, 36, 38, 53–55, 59, 61, 63–64, 74, 82, 100, 127
    risk factors, 35, 38, 114
    symptoms, 35
    treatment, 36–38
    types, 35
contact lenses, 25, 40

diabetes, 31, 45, 62, 64, 86–87, 95
dry eye syndrome (ocular surface disease), 21, 42
    causes, 40, 42
    control & prevention with diet, 40, 42, 74, 106
    definition, 39, 42
    diagnosis, 40
    symptoms, 39, 42
    treatment, 40–42

East-Indian cuisine, 104
eggs, 52, 59, 86–87, 132, 134
environmental factors in eye disease, 19, 24, 40, 42–43, 53
exercise & physical activity, 20, 32, 113, 122–123, 127, 136
eye examination, 27–28, 36, 44
eyelid disorders (blepharitis and meibomianitis)
    causes, 43, 46
    definition, 43, 46
    diagnosis, 44
    effects, 43
    control & prevention with diet, 44, 46

    symptoms, 43
    treatment, 44, 46

farmers' markets, 72, 80
fats & fat intake, 59, 82, 87, 93, 97, 104, 109–110
fiber, 34, 49, 52, 70, 79, 80, 84, 88
    definition, 62
    and eye disease, 63, 101
    and general health, 64, 101
    recommended intake, 63, 129
    sources, 63, 95, 101, 104, 106
fish, 21, 32, 40–41, 52, 56–58, 74–77, 81, 92, 105–106, 129, 131–132
    mackerel 58, 74, 76–77, 132
    mercury content in, 58, 75, 76
    rainbow trout, 58, 74, 76–77, 132
    salmon, wild, 21, 58, 74–77, 93, 132
    sardines, 21, 58, 74–77, 132
    tuna, 40, 58, 74–77, 83, 92, 132
flax seed, 21, 56–58, 86, 95, 102, 106–107, 133
    oil, 40, 42, 57–58, 106–107, 109,
    smoothie recipe, 107
flavonoids, 139
fruit, 21, 52–55, 59, 61, 72, 80, 84–85, 88–91, 102, 131, 133–134
    apricots, 85, 88–89, 98, 102, 133
    avocado, 88–91, 100, 133
    berries, 63, 87–88, 91, 102, 107
    cantaloupe, 88–91, 107, 133
    citrus, 63, 72, 88,
    fruit salad recipe, 91
    kiwi, 88–91, 133

glare, 35, 116–119
glasses (corrective lenses), 26, 37–38, 118
glycemic index & glycemic load, 33, 38, 49, 63, 100–101
    definition, 64
    and eye disease, 64
    and general health, 64
green vegetables, 54, 70, 84–85, 132, 134
    broccoli, 84–85, 132
    Brussels sprouts, 63, 84–85, 132
    green beans, 84–85
    peas, 84–85, 132

Index

Health Canada, 51, 58, 76, 120–121, 128, 136
Heart and Stroke Foundation, 63, 128

immune system, 45, 53, 56, 59–60
inflammation, 25, 42–46, 56
Institute of Medicine (USA), 51, 54, 61

leafy green vegetables, 54, 70–73, 131–132
    arugula, 70, 72
    dandelion greens, 70-71, 132
    kale, 70–72, 132
    lettuce, 70–72, 132
    radicchio, 70, 72, 87, 132
    rapini, 70, 72
    salad dressing recipe, 111
    spinach, 70–73, 83, 87, 132
lifestyle, effect on eye-health, 20, 25, 31, 33, 45, 113–123, 127–130, 136, 138–139
lutein & zeaxanthin (carotenoids), 21, 32, 49, 52–53, 70–71, 74, 79, 82–84, 86–89
    definition, 54
    and eye disease, 55, 114
    and general health, 55
    recommended intake, 54, 129

meal ideas, 72, 77, 81, 83, 85, 87, 91, 93, 98, 102, 105, 107
Mediterranean cuisine, 71, 75, 104
Mexican cuisine, 104

North American diet, 44–45, 60, 76
nutraceuticals, 19
nuts and seeds, 52, 56–57, 59–60, 95–98, 105, 131, 133–134
    almonds, 95–98
    cashews, 95, 97–98
    eyefoods nut mix recipe, 98
    hazelnuts, 95
    nut butters, 97–98
    pecans, 95
    pine nuts, 95, 98
    pistachios, 95
    pumpkin seeds, 95, 97–98
    soybeans (edamame), 95
    sunflower seeds, 95, 97
    walnuts, 58, 72, 85, 95, 97–98

oil, 40, 42, 52, 54, 56–59, 72–73, 82, 85, 107, 109–111, 131, 133–134
    canola oil, 58, 109–11, 133
    flax seed oil
    olive oil, 72–73, 77, 81, 85, 98, 105, 109–111, 133–134
    salad dressing recipe, 111,
    walnut oil, 109–110, 58, 73, 85
omega-3 fatty acids, 21, 32–34, 36, 38, 40-42, 44–46, 74, 76, 86, 88–89, 92, 95, 97, 104–106, 109, 129, 132,
    definition, 56
    and eye disease, 57
    and general health, 57
    omega-6 to omega-3 ratio, 40, 45, 57–58
    recommended intake, 57
    types, 56, 58
orange peppers, 54, 82–83, 87, 105, 132, 134
orange vegetables, 79–81, 134
    carrots, 79–81, 107, 132, 134;
    carrot fries recipe, 81
    pumpkin, 79–81; pumpkin seeds, 95, 97–98, 132
    sweet potato, 61, 79–81, 132
    squash, 79–81, 132
oxidation, 53, 96
oysters, 60, 92–93

protein, 33, 74,77, 86, 92, 98, 104, 131, 133–134

recipes
    carrot fries, 81
    eyefoods basic salad dressing, 111
    eyefoods smoothie with flax seed, 107
    eyefoods nut mix, 98
    fruit salad, 91
    whole grain cooking times, 103
resveratrol, 138–139
retina, 29, 31, 33, 54, 114–115, 139

seafood, 52, 60, 92–93
smoking, effect on eye-health, 20, 31, 33–34, 45, 53, 113, 120, 122–123, 127, 136
sunglasses as UV protection, 20, 33, 37, 114–119, 136
    photochromic lenses 117–118
    polarized lenses, 116–117

turkey, 81, 83, 92–93, 133

UV light, 31, 35, 38, 53, 62, 113–119

vision problems (also refractive error), 20, 25, 28
Vitamin C (ascorbic acid), 21, 32, 52, 53, 59, 70–71, 79, 82–83, 84, 88–89
    definition, 55
    and eye disease, 55
    and general health, 56
    recommended intake, 55, 129
Vitamin D, 74
    definition, 62
    and eye disease, 62
    and general health, 62
    recommended intake, 62
Vitamin E, 21, 32, 52–53, 70, 74–75, 79, 82–84, 86, 88, 92, 95, 97, 100, 106, 109–110, 129
    definition, 59
    and eye disease, 59
    and general health, 59
    recommended intake, 59
vitamin supplements, 32–34, 49, 50, 54, 56, 59, 60–62, 79

weekly nutrition targets, 20, 70, 74, 79, 82, 84, 86, 88, 92, 95, 100, 104, 106, 109, 128
whole grains, 21, 34, 52, 64, 87, 93, 100–103, 131, 133
    barley, 63–64, 85, 100–103
    bran cereal, 62, 100–102, 133
    bread, 63–64, 93, 98, 100, 102, 131
    bulgur, 101, 103
    cooking times for whole grains, 103
    oatmeal, 63, 91, 100–102, 107, 133
    pasta, 93, 98, 100–101, 103
    quinoa, 101, 103
    wheat berries, 101, 103
World Health Organization (WHO), 121

zinc, 31–32, 52, 70, 79, 86, 88–89, 92–93, 95, 97, 106
    definition, 60
    and eye health, 60
    and general health, 60
    recommended intake, 60, 129–130